T0146638

UNDERSTANDING THE DENTIST

ISHMAEL BRUCE

BSc; DDS(Dal); DDPH; MSc(Toronto); FGCS (Ghana)

authorHOUSE®

AuthorHouse™
1663 Liberty Drive
Bloomington, IN 47403
www.authorhouse.com
Phone: 1 (800) 839-8640

Published by AuthorHouse 10/12/2017

ISBN: 978-1-5462-0558-6 (sc)
ISBN: 978-1-5462-0556-2 (hc)
ISBN: 978-1-5462-0557-9 (e)

Library of Congress Control Number: 2017913058

Print information available on the last page.

Any people depicted in stock imagery provided by Thinkstock are models, and such images are being used for illustrative purposes only. Certain stock imagery © Thinkstock.

This book is printed on acid-free paper.

—How to beat bad breath
—Do your gums bleed when you brush?
—Should baby teeth be fixed?
—Does my child need braces?
—What are sealants and do they work
—Can the dentist treat his own wife?

CONTENTS

PREFACE

This quotation appeared in the November 1994 publication of the Canadian Dental Association Journal:

"the Canadian Dental Association, in partnership with the Canadian Public Health Association and a group of other national health associations, was participating in an across Canada literacy campaign on health literacy and the impact it may have on a client's health, and to promote the availability of materials in plain language to facilitate the process. Tests have shown that patient compliance can increase by about as much as 50 per cent if you speak and provide information in plain language". This report, although written in the 90s and in Canada, has a recurring theme and applies to this day not just in Canada but all around the globe.

By definition health literacy is the degree to which individuals have **the capacity to obtain,** process and understand basic health information and services needed to make appropriate health decisions. To have the capacity to obtain health information means **the information should be readily available to the individual.**

This book has therefore been prepared with just such an urgency in mind.

ABOUT THE DENTIST

You may have read it somewhere, and it is true; according to the American Dental Association's Bureau of Economic Research and Statistics, suicide rates among dentists are almost double those of other professionals. Dentists, aside of sustaining the ever present lower back-problem, most often go on disability for reasons of mental or nervous problems.

All these observations, probably with the exception of the unavoidable postural and ergonomic work-related back problem, are undoubtedly stress-related. The dentist, for reasons not hitherto revealed, is one professional under great pressure. "There is tremendous pressure, as soon as you graduate, to keep your head down and go like crazy until basically something breaks," notes one 1994 Canadian Dental Association Communique which is still applicable, if not even more acute. The end-result of this 'workaholic sprint' is an individual who feels too guilty to take a few days off, much less a badly needed vacation. For those who may not understand where this pressure to achieve comes from, it is because by the time the dental student has graduated from the Dental School, he or she would be in debt for at least Four Hundred Thousand Dollars ($400,000). Although this scenario is definitely true in the industrially developed countries, it is beginning to now apply also to the developing countries where up till this point dental education has been free through respective government grants.

One of the reasons for the stress is that dentistry is, in many ways, a trap. Those who choose to be dentists are often high achievers and are driven, caring individuals. Perfection, status and accomplishment are important to them, although these values are also key ingredients of chronic stress.

Another area of anxiety for dentists, is the fact that they never want to quit practicing even when burnt out because they feel they cannot do anything else. This, unfortunately, is self-deception, seeing that dentists have immense potential for other arenas of entrepreneurship. A dentist, as an employer and a team leader, can enter into areas where leadership is required. He may enter the investment field or else into management where his expertise as a business person will come handy. With his experience as a people's person, his organizational acumen can be tapped in other areas. And he can even be a President, with his business acumen, like the Trump!

But ask any dentist and he will tell you there is nothing after dentistry, which is indeed a shame. Dentists are a crazy bunch indeed!

Unfortunately, many in the healing professions —dentistry and medicine, in particular —give of themselves at the expense of not meeting their own needs. Another observation not well-known and not stressed enough, is the fact that highly driven people, such as dentists, often suffer from a deficiency of self-esteem, which can leave them with poor communication skills. Consequently, many dentists often feel uncomfortable interacting with patients or staff, and have difficulty being assertive or playing the role of the boss. Such individuals, expecting perfection and accomplishment often get into dentistry, into this very demanding job where a lot of skill is required and one's stamina, focus and concentration are sorely tested.

In dentistry, more than probably any other profession, there are innumerable demands, not only in doing clinical work, but also in dealing with people and running a business. "From the moment they graduate, dentists come under the great deal of financial pressure that can last for years." Again, this will soon be a reality even in developing countries, where most hitherto have been government employed and are on salary. In many of these developing countries the cash-strapped governments cannot employ the increasing number of new graduates like they used to and many new graduates are therefore presently under-utilized and are leaving to other countries, of course usually to the developed countries. This scenario is now causing a brain drain of the worse kind. Worse kind because these young professionals are the individuals most needed in these developing countries for nation building.

One of the serious side effects of stress, unfortunately, is substance abuse, and because drugs are relatively easy for them to access, dentists, like physicians, supposedly have one of the highest rates of drug and alcohol abuse.

Here, then, is the profile of the dentist. Probably not all dentists answer to these descriptions but most probably do. The unfortunate realization is that dentists are such private and introspective bunch of hard-workers that many, while appreciating these problems quietly within, will deny them in public for fear of appearing weak.

I often ask myself this rhetoric question: Are we (dentists) all crazy before we get into dentistry or do we get crazy while in dental school? No one has been able to answer my question yet! And even I cannot answer the question. I am crazy now, as a dentist, but was I crazy before I entered Dental School? No idea, but even if I knew the answer, I would at this point take the Fifth.

INTRODUCTION

So you are going to the dentist. There is a tooth that has been bothering you for weeks and you've now mustered enough courage to have it fixed. Or you think you might need some denture work (false teeth or ``falsies). Or you are visiting for a check-up and cleaning. How do you prepare for these visits? To most people dentistry is a necessary evil and it seems to me this is so because the rationales and the diagnostics as well as the treatment procedures of the profession are not as well known. Medicine has done a better job at educating the consuming populace to understand a reasonable amount of their personal disease entities and how best to care for these problems.

For example, there are many self-help books and other publications on Medicine for the layman whereas I don't find any on dentistry, with the exception of the odd entries in Reader's Digest, the odd magazine or in some newspaper on some sensational procedures like bleaching or implants. Otherwise there are none or very few general reference publications on Dentistry for the patient.

In my 45 years of practicing dentistry, I have realized that the majority of people going to the dentist are poorly prepared for these visits. Most people do not know that dentists need their (the patients') input to provide an effective and satisfying treatment plan and outcomes. It seems as if most people have abrogated the care of their own bodies to the whim of the dentist and yet, they complain incessantly of the treatment given. For example, how can an adult go to the dentist without first cleaning the mouth and teeth and go with all the crud from breakfast or lunch still on the teeth? I feel a patient should at least brush the teeth before the dental appointment. It is like going for a medical check-up and not showering first. And how can an adult, with several large and open rotten cavities all over the mouth, with some already abscessed (infected), come in to see the dentist, sit in the chair and without any remorse point to the tiny insignificant little chip on the corner of the front tooth? Oh, sure, this tiny chip might be significant all right to the patient but it also shows poor prioritization and is like spitting on a wildfire.

I always cringe whenever a patient comes to my office and after some questioning from me about their dental health to be told, "You are the doctor or the expert. You should know what to do``. Some cop out! The fact that quite a number of patients who come to see me in my clinic, and I am sure to other offices, continuously recount incidents of some reputedly 'bad treatment' given them by a previous dentist indicates that there is a problem here and something has got to be done. Most of dentists' problems arise from communication obfuscation. And we think it is only with our teenagers that we have such problems! In fact, most people will find a derogatory comment to make with respect to some dentist or the treatment received sometime in their life from another dentist, if asked, and sometimes even when not asked, it is offered rather willingly.

This book is designed therefore to provide you the patient with the right information so you know the right questions to ask at the dentist's. It is with the intention of imparting information to the public, the kind of information that up till now has been held hostage within the dental profession, so that even before the dental visit eventually occurs that you the patient will have an idea of what will probably happen at that visit. The book will also be useful to the dental student and new dentists who will find that there are certain things they will not learn from Dental School. A lot of the tips that come only with practice and experience will be presented here.

It has been written as a quick read and in a simplified language so everyone will understand. Wherever necessary each technical term has been explained (in parentheses) so you don't have to stop and search for the meaning.

Before a dental visit, find the Chapters that deal with your particular problem, read them through and acquaint yourself with the pertinent information. The objective here is to eliminate all surprises and the unknown, to reinforce or correct what general impressions you may have of certain dental procedures and their possible outcomes, and to put you in the proper frame of mind so that both you and the dental office will enter into a more amicable relationship throughout the period of treatment.

A dental practice should never be a place of antagonism and acrimony. It is such a close relationship physically that any misunderstanding, if not straightened out at the outset, presents a mental and stressful chasm which persists throughout that relationship. When such a chasm is allowed to exist there is a lose-lose situation and the problem is finally resolved either by the patient eventually leaving the practice and going to another dentist or the dentist decides he has had enough and refuses to see the patient.

It is funny but as a dentist, I have always likened the relationship with the dentist to that of a marital relationship. It is different in the case of one's relationship with the physician in the sense that most people spend only a few effective minutes with the physician – at the most ten minutes per visit whereas it runs into an average of about thirty minutes with the dentist. Because the dentist actually performs a surgical procedure at most every visit of each patient (except in cases of consultations and examinations), more intensive time is spent at very close quarters with patients. Throughout each of these surgical procedures the attention of the dentist is solely focused on the patient whose every twitch and nuance is clearly registered on the dentist's psyche. Under this circumstance it is paramount that the minds should meet. The meeting of the mind's engender empathy and a serenity in the focus of the dentist so that the work goes on smoothly and with great care.

It is stressed that there cannot and should not be any adversarial feelings between the care-giver, the dentist, and you the patient. It is a most unsettling and uncomfortable feeling for the dentist, and I am sure for the patient as well, being that close to one another physically and knowing that there is a lingering distrust for one another. Isn't this similar to a marital relationship? It is in this light that this book has been written —to provide a more harmonious relationship in the service of dental care. And so that it will be easily and quickly read it has been done in fewer pages than it normally would have been for a subject of this magnitude so that one could complete it in a very short time so as to leave one with enough time for the oncoming visit. And before anyone accuses me of sexual discrimination, I must right here and now mention that of course I know there are male as well as female dentists. However, in most places in the book the 'dentist' has been referred to with the pronoun, –him–. This is not an oversight — it is for want of a single, more appropriate word to represent both sexes. I just got tired writing – he/she – repeatedly so I decided to go with only one designation. Believe it or not, and as a research dental professional, I tossed and the males won. So there. And I could be wrong but I think at the present, anyway, and in North America, for sure, there are more male dentists than females? No? Ah well….c'est la vie!

CHAPTER 1

PREVALENT HORROR STORIES ABOUT DENTISTS

There are as many horror stories about dentists as there are dentists. We seem to be the only professionals who are always told, right in our faces to boot, that we are disliked. It has in fact become the opening conversational piece in many dental offices. A lady, or a man, walks reluctantly into the operatory (dental office), looks around for a place to sit, although there is only one obvious chair for her to sit on (many times I have come into the operatory with a patient sitting on either my chair or the assistant's chair!). Of course the assistant should seat the patient, technically, but I have seen places where the assistant just takes the patient to the door of the operatory and asks the patient 'to sit in the chair' without indicating which of the three chairs in the room is for her. Finally the patient gets to sit, reluctantly and hesitatingly, in the appropriate seat in the patient's chair, and the first sentence she utters is: "I must tell you I hate dentists." And as if an after-thought, she quickly adds, "but it's not you personally." I have heard this so so many times that even though I think I understand, that it is just a crying out for help –'please, pretty please, don't hurt me', I still, after all these years, feel a little flicker of guilt and anguish when I hear it.

And then there are the men who, although will say this in a jocular manner, really mean the same thing by the humorous remark: "we don't want to hurt each other, do we now!" In my many years of practice, I have come to rationalize these utterances, rightly or wrongly, as coming from people who are primarily apprehensive and anxious about the impending surgery and really do not mean any harm. What I have always wondered, however, is what lasting effects these remarks have in the long run on the psyche of dentists who are bombarded with this jocular but subliminal debilitating verbal abuse every day. No one has done any studies to verify this but do these remarks, for example, have any connection with the observed fact that dentists are reputed to have the highest suicide rates among all professionals? And you still wonder why dentists are nuts, huh?

But probably the most prevalent horror story about dentists is the one about drilling teeth with inadequate freezing. I have heard these anecdotes so many times that now I listen to them without actually 'hearing' them, you know, where you are listening, but you are not there? Almost every patient has a story of the dentist who insisted on doing a filling without enough freezing. It is probably not an exaggeration to say that dentistry has changed a whole lot in the last thirty years. But have freezing techniques changed that much? The reason I am usually rather skeptical about all these accusations is that I am a lot older than many of these complainants so it is not that long ago when they must have had their dental work done, even as children. And I learnt what freezing technique I presently use about fourty something years ago and it still seems to be pretty adequate, from all accounts. It all seems to boil down not to the era but generally to impatient and rushed dentists, if all these accusations are true. But true or not, what I gather from these comments in my own work is for me to be as caring as I can and to the best of my abilities provide the needed treatment as comfortably and as painlessly as I know how.

I believe a patient should be able to draw the dentist's attention to the fact that the freezing is not enough. I feel it is just human and good sense to acknowledge the patient's feelings. In fact it is mandatory in my office "to let me know if the freezing is not deep enough so that I can add a little bit more to make it comfortable." Funny, but every time I have said this at the beginning of the work, which is with every surgical patient, I have always chuckled to myself, being constantly reminded of the announcement made on commercial airlines by the flight captains just before the flight. It has become so repetitious to the point now that

I plan to record my instructions and have the assistant play it just before I start the surgery. "Lady (or gentleman), please fasten your seat belt. Your dentist today is Dr. T.F. (Tooth Fairy) Bruce. At any time, while I am working, if you find you need a little more freezing please don't hesitate to put your right hand up and I will stop to add a little more freezing to make you comfortable, (as if 'comfortable' can be used to describe a dental experience!) And by the way, have a nice day." This information is for me just as much as for the patient because somehow, personally, I am not able to perform as fast and as efficiently if I suspect that the freezing is inadequate. Usually, the body language of the patient in the chair will tell me if a little bit more freezing is warranted. And then if at that juncture, when I stop to add more freezing, the patient feels everything is fine, he will let me know. Moreover, I almost always enter into an agreement with each patient to put the right hand up (so that if they have any inclination to hit, I can stop them. I have a reason to my madness and I am also right-handed, I'll have you know); but it's a simple way to empower patients to signal me to stop whenever there is the need for more freezing. And I must tell my fellow dentists that adding more freezing to make sure the patient is comfortable does not mean you are incompetent. It just makes good surgical sense.

It does not work that well with my child patients, however, or I should say it works too well with them, and I am presently looking for a better way to let the child patients understand to let me know at any time if more freezing is needed by raising the right hand. So far, every time I have given this instruction to a child patient the child immediately shoots a hand up as if to see if I really mean what I said. And coming to think of it, the child is right. Didn't I say "at any time"? And they figure right at the beginning is as good a time as any. Funny, kids. The other problem is that the hand comes up very frequently throughout the procedure, at the slightest hint of even a detectable change in the pitch of the drill. You stop and ask them if they need more freezing, and a lot of times the answer, with a very straight face, is No! with a sideways shake of the head.

But I have also come to the conclusion that many dental visits are or were not as horrible as people have painted the occasions to be. In a lot of cases the patient gives you horror stories abound in the marketplace about dentists, only to 'sensitize' the dentist to their impending situation. One person says this, and this person says it to another person and before you know it the harmless incident has been so embellished and is now such a horror story.

Like, for example in this incident. The dentist has just finished taking five badly decayed teeth on the same side of the mouth out of a 45 year old man. As the gentleman walks back into the reception area, a nosy acquaintance waiting her turn turns around and inquisitively asks:

"What did you have done?"

"I had five teeth removed," replied our friendly neighbour.

"Boy, that must hurt!," offered the nosy 'friend'.

"Actually, no it didn't hurt at all." Calmly, the gentlemen, without malice, this time really deflates her balloon. "You know, that has never bothered me!"

Good for you! You see, some people always have to appear more knowledgeable than others when it comes to this dental thing. But what these rumour mongers, like our nosy neighbour, have to remember is that not everyone experiences events the same way they do. To some people, dentistry, believe it or not, offers a very beautiful experience. I know people who have conditioned themselves to liken the vibration of the slow-speed drill to the calming effect of a vibrating pillow and therefore don't find it annoying at all. In fact, it makes them snooze off. So you see, forcing your personalized, embellished and prejudicial opinions on others may prove disastrous on your frail ego if you tango with the wrong person. And the more you do this the more you reveal some notions which others around you may come to find boring and controlling should their experience happen to be in fact complimentary and positive.

The bad news is that only the few incidents of bad treatment at the hands of a few dentists get rumoured around. The good news is that I also know that good dentistry also gets rumoured around, so there is hope for dentists yet to recover from years of bad publicity.

Dentistry has changed and is still changing. Dentists are, in my opinion, very compassionate people trying to do what they can to alleviate pain. But many people, even when subsequent experiences happen to be painless, cannot believe their luck and will still adhere to their first impressions (because they cannot believe it can be so good an experience) and therefore deny themselves and others the enjoyment of a beautiful experience.

CHAPTER 2

MAKING THE APPOINTMENT

One of the nightmares of the dental receptionist is the patient on the phone who wants to know what a dental filling costs. It is impossible to answer this question without first going into the whole dental anatomy of the tooth. The receptionist cannot answer this question because the dental fees for fillings depend on many factors. Let's go through one incident for you to see what I am talking about.

Krr—krrr—krrr

RECEPTIONIST: Hello! Dr. T. F's office! (from here on we will use Dr. T.F. for Dr. Bruce)

PATIENT: I would like to have a tooth filled – could you tell me how much it will cost to fix it?

RECEPTIONIST: (eh, pausing with frustration in her voice) – Maam, it is difficult to give you a quote. Would you like to come in for the dentist to see you first? (a big sigh but off the record–)

PATIENT; (impatient) all I want is just one filling (Little does she know! Now here we go—)

RECEPTIONIST: Ok, Maam, is it a front tooth or a back tooth? (The receptionist hears the patient muttering something like –What?—in the background so she goes on to explain)—I mean, is the tooth you want to have fixed in the front or in the back of the mouth.?

PATIENT: Oh, I don't know – it is one of the back teeth —eh, in the middle, I think. Wait, let me see. (After what seems like ages) – it is one of the smaller back teeth in the middle, yes.

RECEPTIONIST: (wondering whether the patient is in the bathroom looking in the mirror or just peeking through her compact mirror) – Maam, on which surface or side of the tooth is the cavity?

PATIENT: The surface – what do you mean? And cavity, you mean the chip on my tooth, what cavity?

RECEPTIONIST: (almost thinking out loud) I mean, is the hole on top or on the side of the tooth?

PATIENT: There is a big hole on the top and my tongue keeps getting at it. My tongue is all raw from rubbing it.

RECEPTIONIST: — (fighting the urge to tell Maam to get her blasted tongue out where it does not belong – you can't control your tongue, can you? She takes a deep breath as she has been taught to do in times like this and manages to add –.) Does the hole involve only one or two surfaces of the tooth? –(now trying to compose herself)—sometimes it may appear like it is on only one surface but it may involve another surface in which case the fee is for two surfaces.

PATIENT: Oh, I see.

RECEPTIONIST: Now, do you want a white filling or a grey filling?

By this time, I am sure the patient would have already hung up the phone and probably gone to another dental office. But to reach a specific quote of a fee for any specific filling on a tooth the receptionist and the dentist have to consider all these variables. The easiest way is to make an appointment for consultation at which time a specific examination will be done and a fee quoted.

The Emergency Appointment

Because of time constraint, most dentists will generally restrict an emergency appointment to just what it says –an emergency visit. All too often a patient will show up for an emergency appointment but then will decide unilaterally that whilst he is in the chair that the dentist should do this tooth and then that tooth all in that one appointment. Much as most dentists that I know would like to do everything the individual may need done (after all he is making more money by doing so) many factors may prevent him from obliging the patient.

This ruse is particularly employed by individuals who have stayed away from the dentist for years and now have to go because some teeth have 'bombed out' (rotten away) and now need treatment in a bad way. Other times it is the patient who admits to you he is so petrified of dentists (read, "dental treatment") that he wants everything done all today, now that 'you've got me in the chair.'

One of the problems with some dental emergencies is that the status of the tooth may in fact preclude a more definitive treatment at the time it is presented. The dentist may need at this stage to provide a palliative (soothing) treatment for now and put the tooth on observation for a prescribed period before a more definitive treatment can be scheduled. Of course there will be a fee charged for this phase of the treatment as well as when the final treatment is provided.

Then consideration has to be given to those people who have already made their regular appointments. In many busy offices an emergency appointment is usually sandwiched between regular appointments. It is therefore not fair to let the legitimate appointment wait and wait while the emergency appointment stretches into hours. In my office all emergencies are advised that I will have time to alleviate the pain; if there is more time, however, sure, we can do more work.

There have been instances where it would also have served both the emergency patient and myself well to have kept strictly to this emergency rule. There have been some occasions where a patient suffering with an excruciating acute phase of an abscess, should have been given antibiotics and dismissed to go home for about a week or so before returning for the extraction. With empathy and an obvious appreciation of the situation I had gone ahead in many of these situations to freeze the tooth and ready it for extraction only to find that all attempts at the freezing (the tooth) ended up inadequate. I don't know how other dentists feel but I have always felt very frustrated and disappointed (not mentioning the patient's) when all attempts at freezing a tooth fail. One redeeming aspect though is that all that freezing helps reduce the pain from the bad tooth so at least the patient is a little more comfortable than when he came in. But it still does not solve the underlying problem.

Dentists, typical surgeons than they are, are often reluctant to leave a tooth alone and allow the situation to resolve reasonably with a prescription before putting the forceps to the tooth. And they cannot be blamed because patients always expect a dentist 'to do something' at each visit. But then, surgeons have always been blamed for being scalpel happy anyway. And you feel like you have not done enough for the patient who has come to you seeking relief. It appears that in dental surgery you really do not spell 'relief' with a prescription! In dentistry, you give real relief only when you've done the surgery for relief of the pain. Many a time a prescription is met with the retort — "is that all?" or "You are not doing anything today?" As if the last 10 minutes spent looking in the mouth and planning the treatment was "nothing".

Toothaches And Self-Examination

In many cases the offending tooth at a toothache appointment can be easily identified. In some cases, however, the patient is not able to identify which tooth is causing the problem. It is a widely-observed truism, as most patients and dentists alike will well attest, that toothaches have a notorious reputation of vanishing just when the patient presents at the dentist. This particular tooth may have been bothering the dickens out of the patient for days but just when the patient shows at the dental office the tooth with the ache takes the fifth amendment and decides to cool it! Of course sometimes the patient would have taken some pain-killers prior to the appointment and that helps sooth the tooth some.

Unless there is an obviously cracked tooth or filling or a fully blown abscess the dentist may not be able to identify the exact offending tooth. Although there are other reasons for a toothache, some toothaches may not present any observable sequel (pathology, disease) to aid in the diagnosis. Under these circumstances the patient may be sent home maybe with some pain-killers to wait until something concrete shows up. It will therefore help if the individual attempts to identify the problematic tooth before-hand at home by looking in the mirror and examining the area in the mouth. One way of doing this is by pressing on each tooth in the area from the top, and from all sides, with one's fingers to determine if any of the manipulations elicit any pain.

One should also make a mental note whether temperature has any effect on the tooth.

1.   Does the tooth react to hot foods like tea, coffee, pizza, fried plantain?
2.   Does it react to cold foods like ice cream, cold water, cold beer?
3.   If any of these temperature changes elicit a noticeable pain does this sensation last a long time or does it peter off when the stimulus (the offending food or drink) is removed?
4.   Do both hot and cold stuffs bother the tooth?
5.   Does cold help take away the pain? Do you find that putting ice-cold items on the tooth soothe it?

     Other tests that you can do yourself to help expedite or reach a valid diagnosis are:

6.   Does the tooth react to sweets like chewing gum, chocolates, or fried hot plantain?
7.   Does biting on the tooth hurt and does it only hurt when you bite on it?
8.   Does pressing on the tooth relieve the pain?
9.   Does the tooth "feel long", like it has moved higher out of its socket (its bony encasement; each tooth sits in a cradle of bone)?
10. Do you presently have a cold or the flu? Any sinus problem recently?

     Making a note of these effects on the tooth will make it very easy for the dentist to come to a proper diagnosis and provide the appropriate treatment in the shortest possible time.

     The type of pain is also very helpful:

11. Is it a throbbing pain, a sharp or a low-grade, dull, nagging ache?

12. Does a change in posture make a difference? Is the pain aggravated by lying down? Does it throb when you change posture, or positions?

Personally identifying all these affective parameters impacting on the tooth at home will enable the dentist to come to a more conclusive diagnosis even when the pain is gone at the time of the appointment.

I truly believe the philosopher who said "happiness is the absence of pain." Human beings will do anything to attain that elusive sate of happiness. A toothache is one event that easily comes to mind that makes even the 'coward' courageous. It is a shame every dentist does not have a sign in front of his office- IN PURSUIT OF HAPPINESS.

Weekend Emergencies

Many individuals, I am sure, have had the misfortune of having a filling (in a filled tooth) break or fall out at a most inopportune time. Because of the high prevalence of this occurrence I thought of patenting a preparation some years back for public use for such emergencies. But it appears somebody heard me and scooped the idea because for a few years now, I have seen on television a preparation 'new' on the market for just such emergency. I said 'new' because although dentists have always had this medication for office use it has not been publicized or made available to the public in the drug stores. The medication consists of a powder and a liquid. These are mixed and simply inserted into the hole (cavity left by the lost or fractured filling) with the fingers.

Up till now, almost anything has been used to stop the pain – anything that will physically block the hole to prevent food from impacting. The home-made 'fillings' have ranged from chewing gum, mud, cow dung, cotton pellet, ground cloves, to aspirins placed in or around the offending tooth. Aspirin is used quite often, the only problem being that if used over a long period of time, like ten days, it leaves an 'aspirin burn' around the gums. It is not so much the time factor with the aspirin but the placement—it will not cause acid burn if the aspirin is confined

INSIDE the hole IN the tooth. The advice is this — go to the dentist at the first sign of a toothache. Better yet, why not make it a habit to see the dentist every six months or yearly, pain or no pain, before a toothache. You don't necessarily have to do this every 3 or 6 months, but you can visit at intervals that suit you and will not be long enough to allow a small hole in the tooth get bigger and bother you.

CHAPTER 3

CONSULTATION AND EXAMINATION

CHILDREN

Parents are always wondering when is the right age to take a child to the dentist. Children, in short, should be seen when they have to be seen, with no age limitations. No child is too young to have the teeth checked as long as there is a tooth in the mouth. I have always asked parents to bring their children in for a check-up once teeth appear in the mouth.

In most practices, however, children are seen for their first dental visitation at about the age of three. This schedule, really, should be for the children who up till this point have not had any indication of a dental disease or problem and everything since has seemed 'normal' to the parents. Recent guideline has it that kids should be seen when the first teeth come in (after about the sixth month), or within six months of the eruption of the first tooth or close to around a year old.

However, some children may have to be seen earlier than that and may have to have their initial visit even before the age of one. I have seen children as early as six months in my practice. Little children with teething problems may be seen early if they won't eat as a result of teething pains. And then, there are those who have rampant caries (lots of 'cavities') and will need attention at any age where this becomes obvious. Especially in the case of Early Caries Syndrome (ECC), also sometimes called nursing caries syndrome (toddlers with lots of 'cavities' resulting directly or indirectly from poor feeding habits), some of these children (usually between the ages of 2 and 5) will need surgery if multiple abscesses (painful 'gum-boils') are developed. I have had kids referred for surgery to have four front teeth removed and four back teeth filled at the age of 18 months. In fact Early Childhood Caries (ECC) account for about one-third of all day surgeries performed on Canadian children between the ages of 1 and 5, according to a study by the Canadian Institute for Health Information (website: cihi.ca). The CIHI report highlights the prevalence of oral health neglect in Canadian children and raises awareness of a health care issue that can be avoided.

But the onus is on the parents to check the child's teeth everyday as the teeth are cleaned to make sure no disease or abnormality goes undetected or unattended. If a parent sees any suspicious discoloration on a tooth, and is not sure what it is, then it should be checked by the dentist. A few parents will retort, "the child does not allow me to clean or look in the mouth". I feel it is negligence if the parent watches over a child from birth until the child develops abscesses at age 18 months. Would you rather the child develop gum-boils and we have to now force open the child's mouth to take the teeth out at age 18 months? This is not hearsay, I have seen and referred several of such cases for hospital general anaesthesia work.

Nursing Caries Syndrome

This is a condition all too familiar in the very young children usually from around the age of 16 months to two and a half years old. These children contract multiple cavities most characteristically in the top front teeth. This can get so serious that sometimes there is nothing left but black stumps where the front teeth used to be — all teeth would have decayed or rotten right to the gums. The older children (over 2 years)would have rotten back teeth as well. If you don't think this is serious check this out:

—-the CIHI report found that each year roughly 19,000 children had dental surgery (a 2-year study), mostly for fillings and extractions (tooth removal) and spent an average of 82 minutes in the operating room under general anaesthesia. Across the country, rates of day surgery operations, expressed as number of operations per 1000 children, ranged from a low of 8.4 to a high of 97.2. The estimated annual hospital related costs totalled $21.2 million, not including costs associated with dental surgeons and anaesthesiologists.

And the cause of this tooth destruction, you may ask? — It is all because, to appease Mary from crying even after her main meal, mother or the care-giver puts sugared water, tea with sugar, fruit juices, or milk in the child's bottle. The bottle is then given to Mary who now happily sucks until she falls asleep, the bottle often left still dangling at the corner of the child's mouth like the inevitable Graucho Marx's cigar. The teeth, awash with stagnant sugared fluids, now provide a fertile feeding ground for the sugar-bugs which get busy at destroying Mary's teeth. And these teeth bugs don't give a hoot whether the warm fertile environment happens to be the 2 year-old Mary or 16 year old Joe.

I understand some parents even go to the extent of actually dipping the child's soother or the teat of the feeding bottle in honey to 'sweeten the pie' for the poor child! The lesson from all this? A child, being put down for the day's nap or for the night, SHOULD NOT be given:

1. the bottle in which there is milk, juice, sweetened-tea or sweetened-water;
2. a soother dipped in sugar, honey or jam;
3. the bottle with the teat dipped in sugar, honey or jam.

Nowadays, mother's breast-milk can be collected and stored for later use. The same precaution applies to this breast-milk, that is, not to be given in the bottle or even fresh and straight from the mother to a sleepy child.

If your child needs the bottle after the main feeding, give only plain water. First, feed the baby with whatever you've made ready, then give the water as the last thing in the bottle. You are in deep poop, of course, if your child does not like water. Kids are smart, and I would too, if your drinking water is as bad as that from my village well. **If that is the case, then the suggestion is to wipe the child's mouth thoroughly after**

feeding with a wet piece of cloth BEFORE the child falls asleep. You may wake the child up momentarily but I would rather that than in the hospital in surgery.

The Care of Your Baby's Mouth

The care of your baby's mouth and teeth should begin immediately after birth and continue, hopefully, for a lifetime. After each feeding (bottle- or breast), your baby's gum pads (when there are no teeth in the mouth yet), should be wiped with a clean damp cloth (like a face towel) to remove any food residue. As the teeth start to appear (from around four to the sixth month), this cleaning process must continue. But make sure to wipe off all food debris from all the chewing surfaces (inside and out) after each feeding. Or follow with a bottle of water. (And, I didn't say a bottle of –beer! Some parents give beer to send a troublesome baby to sleep).

If the plaque and food remnants on the baby's teeth are left uncleaned after each feeding, the risk of tooth decay, yes, even in a sixteen-month old child, is very high. As well, if your baby's teeth are exposed to any form of sugar especially while asleep, the risk of developing early childhood caries (nursing caries syndrome) is also high. And just as in the adult, when the two factors co-exist, that is plaque (or bugs) left on the teeth AND teeth exposed to sugar (whether asleep or awake), the risk of tooth decay is multiplied.

I remember my first encounter with a sixteen-month old boy brought to me because he had developed multiple fistulae (gumboils) **from** the upper front teeth as a result of 'nursing caries syndrome'. At this age there is usually no way any work can be done in the dental chair so I had to remove all his four top front teeth in the hospital under a fast and a light general anesthetic. The problem was that now my little man will not eat because he was missing his front teeth. Eventually, I had to fabricate a very nifty and cute partial denture (false teeth) for him to replace the missing **top** four front teeth. The point here is that no matter how old the child is if he/she develops any 'cavities' then the **teeth** should be taken care of. If the cavities happen to be incipient (small and just beginning) the option might be to keep them under close watch and have them checked every three to four months to make certain they don't get any larger or worse. Hence, if a small black or brown dot is noticed on the surface of any tooth while brushing the child's teeth, and the parent thinks it might be a 'cavity', the thing to do is seek advice from the dentist. And actually, watching these teeth for over 6 months or a year might be too late.

Some Areas of Concern to Parents

One area of concern to most parents is the colour of children's teeth especially when the permanent (adult) front teeth start erupting into the mouth between the ages of five to eight years old. Baby teeth are by nature whiter than the adult permanent teeth that replace them. Hence with the permanent teeth erupting cheek and jowl and just adjacent to the baby teeth, most parents worry about them being "dirty' in comparison with the baby teeth. Of course if the child does not receive good and adequate oral hygiene or does not brush often the teeth may just be that —dirty. However, if there is consistent brushing then the color showing may just be its natural shade. In case of any doubt, particularly where the colour difference appears definitely abnormal, a consultation should be sought at the dentist's to rule out developmental defects.

Another area of concern has to do with the positioning of the now erupting permanent teeth in the front part of the lower jaw when the child is around the age of five to eight years. This stage of dental development, which used to be called 'the ugly duckling stage', probably generates more questions from parents than any other that I can think of. And count me among these worried parents. When one of my **own** daughters exhibited the same crowding problem, guess who was worried? Of course I did not seek a second opinion. How could I (I was supposed to know what to do, right)? Anyway, I had to take my own pill and follow my own advice, which, I am happy to say, proved to be correct. But I learned, since that time, never to take a parent's concern lightly even when the answer may be a very simple one – to me, as the dentist, that is. Now look who is talking! So you see, even we dentists have our own ``teething` problems.

Another area of concern has to do with the same region in the front part of the lower jaw. The baby's lower front teeth are naturally smaller in size compared to the newly erupting permanent teeth replacing them. There is therefore a temporary lack of space for the newly erupting permanent teeth replacing them, especially in the region of the first four teeth in the lower jaw. Parents, take heart, because father nature (there I go again, father nature—sexist, huh,) is so very ordered and here is how. Whereas the front baby teeth in the lower jaw are smaller compared to the new replacement permanent adult front teeth, the back baby molar teeth are usually bigger than the succedaneous (the new, the replacing) permanent back teeth. Hence, it is all naturally arranged perfectly that the lack of space in the lower front jaw is eventually made up, 'all things being equal', by the surplus space realized when the permanent replacement teeth come through in the back of the mouth. (For dental students, what do we call this expected excess space= leeway space)

In about 30% of the cases, though, this spacing problem persists either because of individual hereditary factors or because some baby teeth were prematurely lost previously or were decayed and not fixed and have resulted in a loss of space between the teeth. At this point then, there is a legitimate concern since orthodontic work (braces) may be needed to make more room for the new permanent teeth.

There are, however, times when some baby teeth may have to be removed at this early stage to create room in order to prevent any future crowding of the teeth. But where there is doubt it does not hurt to have a quick consultation visit with the dentist. In cases where your friendly dentist may not be sure of the eventual outcome, he may also then refer you for a quick consultation with the ORTHODONTIST, the dental specialist who deals with braces and proper tooth alignment in the mouth.

What to Tell the Child Patient Before the Appointment

Parents, of course, mean well and try to prepare their children for dental visits in the only way they know how. However, the dental profession has not properly educated or informed parents as to the right way to go about imparting this last minute briefing to their children.

If I was to prepare any of my children for the dentist, (and the need has already arisen, **I must have you know),** I would try not to use certain words like: freezing, pain, needle, hurt, and afraid. All these words have 'fight or flight' connotations, are 'user unfriendly' and invoke an aura of avoidance. There is no doubt in my mind that the use of these 'unfavourable' words by parents, in relation to dental treatments, have conjured in the minds of children some of the unpleasant expectations associated with dental visits. It explains in the main part why many children are spooked even before they enter the dental office.

As a parent, I would try to keep my own anxieties with respect to dental treatments in check at all times but more so when approaching appointment times. Simply put, many parents unknowingly transfer their own fear of dental visits onto the child. It is uncanny how a child will pick up on the parent's mood come dental appointment time. Horror stories about a treatment the parent has had some years back have no place within the earshot of a child, if you want the child to have a more unique and pleasant experience, that is.

The child's dental experience is made or broken by that first dental visit and will be dictated to a large extent by what preparation parents give the child. Some children come into the office all hyped-up and are incessantly shifting every which way, following every little movement of the dentist. These children, right at the outset, are so freaked out that from here on the die is cast for a very unpleasant and unmanageable encounter.

Some parents are so out of it that they will threaten the child with a visit to the dentist and have a tooth removed if the child misbehaved at home. Now how low can you get! As soon as the child associates dentistry with punishment or pain, future dental visits will be shunned like the plaque or looked upon with great trepidation and distrust.

If you cannot find any good things to say about dentistry to the child you will be well-advised to in fact say very little or forever hold your peace and let the dentist do his job. Especially if you do not know much about the subject yourself, then the less you say about it, the better. What the child after all wants to know is 'what the experience is going to be like'. Hence you should make your answers crisp, to the point and without much fanfare. Here is what John probably wants to know the day before the appointment.

"The dentist will count how many new teeth you now have and check them to make sure they are all clean so they don't develop (get) any cavities or holes in them. Holes in the teeth will bother you when you eat. Food gets in the holes and make eating uncomfortable. The dentist is, therefore, a friend who makes sure your teeth are clean. If there are any holes in your teeth when he checks them the dentist will fix them so the teeth will not bother you when you eat. You see, the dentist is our friend and helps us keep our teeth in good shape" If the child asks if it will 'hurt' you should not beat about the bush or try to lie. And do not avoid the question. I feel you should tell the child not how you have experienced it to be but 'how you expect dentistry to be', if you are objective enough. That is, offer an objective view of dental treatment. You could say something like: "The dentist will put your tooth to sleep by rubbing an ointment like Vaseline on your gums next to the tooth that has the hole. The ointment puts your tooth to sleep so that it can be fixed quickly." You may even take a cotton-tipped applicator or Q-Tip, dip it in water and rub it on the gums to show how it will feel. "You see, just like that," you may add. It is even better yet if you have a tube of jiffy. Using that instead of water will numb the gum and show the child how it feels when frozen. "The ointment cleans the tooth and makes the tooth go 'funny' and it goes to sleep. When it feels that way we say the tooth is frozen and it can be fixed without you even knowing it:"

I feel you should not make mention of a 'needle', or a 'shot' or anything that connotes a 'sharp point' or 'pain'. And no reference to the freezing feeling like a 'mosquito bite'. A mosquito bite may not necessarily be reassuring to a child, for that matter even to some adults!

We all have different pain thresholds and your child may probably have one very different from yours.

If the child asks how the hole or 'cavity' is 'fixed', all you need to add is that the dentist will clean the_sugar-bugs out of the tooth with a 'dental spoon' and then will put a filling (NOT medicine!) in the cleaned hole to cover it so food does not get into the tooth and bother you when you eat." I say, 'NOT medicine', because if the child is like some of the kids I have come across, then the mention of medicine will spook him right from the beginning. Some children just hate being given medicine, period—just like some adults I know! The main point here is not to go into all the details of 'drills' and 'machines' and all the dental gadgets. If the dentist is worth his/her salt the child will be introduced to all these gadgets in due course and will explain them in a very easy, patient-friendly manner in order not to arouse any undue apprehension.

ADULTS

In most dental offices, an examination is just what it says, an examination. Unless the dentist says you need cleaning and polishing of the teeth after the examination procedures and YOU demand one, you may not have any cleaning done with the examination. It is therefore up to you to ask for a cleaning, as well, if you want one.

One very common misunderstanding is where the patient walks in and specifically points to a tooth in one area of the mouth as needing some work. Most often this is viewed by the dentist as a specific examination and a complete, thorough examination is not done. Many times these patients have left the office thinking they have had a thorough examination. They, therefore, get very confused when two months down the line, another dental problem develops in the same or a different area of the mouth and they wonder why they should have a problem after they just had a check-up. A specific examination is quite different from a thorough examination and the fee structure reflects that. If you want a thorough or complete check-up with specific attention in any one particular area then say so. I feel some people want to get off paying for a complete check-up with this ruse, but because of time constraints and different billing schedules, most dentists will do just what you ask them to do and will not do any extra work if you asked for a specific examination.

This does not, of course, mean that even though one has just had a complete examination that a dental problem will not arise until your next check-up time. Life is a continuous, dynamic and an unpredictable process and what does not show today may just show up next month. Without doubt you have heard of the individual who died a few weeks after he had his annual medical examination. But then that is life.

To Go or Not To Go, That Is Not the Question

This section is for the adult parent who cannot resist going to the treatment room when the child is taken into the operatory (treatment room).

The parent should be willing to restrain the urge to go into the operatory with the child once the child's turn comes around. It has always surprised me why many parents quickly jump up and follow the child into the operatory. This happens mostly in rural practices, I presume, where everybody knows everybody else in the community and where the dental offices are rather small. But wherever the setting, parents should be trusting enough to believe that the child will be in good hands and allow the dental assistant to walk the child into the treatment room. Hospitals do not allow parents into surgeries for a reason and I do not understand why parents are so eager to want to be in the dental operatory while treatment is going on.

There is the parent who comes into the operatory to 'serve' as the assistant or the assistant's assistant. To be blunt, parents are not an asset to the dentist in the treatment room. When this parent comes in she stands at attention right at the foot of the child just about the edge of the dental chair. The dentist, in the meanwhile, is working away with no problems, so far. The mother sees she is no use around, but keeps her ground, anyway, because she is determined to make her presence felt. She, therefore, decides to be of some use to the dentist by repeating every word the dentist says to the child.

The nuisance may start like this: Dentist to the child: "Can you open your mouth a little bit wider?" The child complies and starts to open the mouth, but before the dentist will say, "Ok, that's fine, now," the mother chimes in; "Dear, the dentist wants you to open your mouth—wide." Lots of times the problem is that the dentist may not want the child to open as WIDE as the mother may think. You see, opening very wide stretches the cheek muscles and prevents an easy access, particularly in the top jaw in the cheek area of the back teeth. Now the dentist has to counteract the mother's untimely intrusion by softly, but almost instantaneously commanding, "not so wide." I can imagine the child's confusion—"I wish these dummies would put their act together and just tell me what they want."

Because I like the children involved in what I am doing and make it fun for them, I usually would ask them to use the suction themselves to suck out the saliva or the water that may have pooled in one area in the mouth. So, I may say to the child, "Could you hold onto this 'straw' and move it around the mouth to suck the water out of your mouth?" No sooner would I have finished the sentence than the mother asks my dental assistant who is right there, on the scene, if I wanted someone else to do the job. And how do you tell this mother that you want the CHILD (patient) to do it and HER out of the way because you don't need her interfering with your technique. Moreover, once you allow her to continue on like this you unwittingly legitimize her presence and then you really have too many cooks on your hands!

Then, there is the 'sneak'. This parent walks into the treatment room immediately after the assistant seats the child, and to the hearing of everyone in the room, the 'snoop' would ask the child—"Do you want mommy here?" –as if that permission is the child's to give! Sure, what five-year old would say "No!" to a loaded question like that! But, here is the revealing part of the whole psychology. There have been many interesting instances where some very independent children have, actually, said no to the mother's request. And what do you think happened? Often, you can almost feel the glare in the mother's scheming eyes as the child, not wanting mom to abandon him, would now recant and recuse herself, shaking the head from side to side. At this point, mom is probably singing in her head---La-la-la-la –laa-la—'mom-gets-to-sta-ay–ay.' All she now needs to complete the coup is to stick her tongue at the dumb-founded staff and say—"I got ya." Yeah, sneaky alright.

In my many years of dental practice, I have found that most children are fine by themselves. For some reason many tend to be more incorrigible in the presence of a parent. What is most annoying is the parent who thinks the dentist needs help with controlling the child and comes to the operatory under the pretense that they are there to help, but help who? If the dentist needs help he will call the parent in. The most disruptive parent is the one who walks uninvited and takes his position alongside the child and decides to repeat whatever the dentist says to the child.

It will start with... "Johnny, don't cry, Dr. Bruce is very good". But who asked you? And 5 year-old Johnny is not even crying, and has not given any sign that he is going to cry. Child now has got the hint that dad is worrying about something.

Dentist... "I am going to wash your tooth with this", dentist squirting a little bit of water out of the tri-flo syringe against the nearest wall to show the child."

Dad, uninvited..."Johnny, Dr. Bruce is going to just wash your tooth."

Dentist..." Johnny, now I am going to wash the tooth so we can fix it and then we will be finished. When I wash it your tooth will start to go to sleep so we can easily fix it.

Dad... "Ya, your tooth will go numb with the freezing and they will use the drill to fix it for you." Now this dad is really here to sabotage my technique. I am getting a little impatient with this patient's dad and my assistant sees through it. What business is it of this man coming to interrupt our work? So my assistant decides to take matters into her own hands and, out of desperation, tells the dad.

"You don't want to stand all throughout the procedure so may be you may want to wait for Johnny in the reception area. Johnny is just fine as you can see. And we will call you as soon as we are finished. It won't take long."

I cringed when my assistant added "it won't take long" because now I am afraid the incorrigible dad would not take the hint and instead say, "Oh then I will stay through it since it won't take long". But this time it worked and dad sauntered out of the operatory, and I bet you mad as hell.

These occurrences have in fact impressed me greatly. The embarrassing part for me, on the other hand, has been many a time where the child is kicking up a storm and the mother is standing next to the child or rubbing the child's arm or legs trying to calm the child down all to no avail. You would think if the parent was any use her presence would calm the child down. But most of the time it doesn't and her presence aggravates the situation.

A Typical Scene Goes Like This:

Child is already quietly sobbing as she sits in the chair. The dentist sits down and addresses Mary (our child parent).

DENTIST: Hi Mary. How old are you? (She spreads four fingers on one hand in front of her face to indicate her age. Children up to about five years old would most always tell you how old they are with their fingers, whether they can speak or not. If their age is more than can be shown on one hand, they will show both hands for you to count the fingers they stick out. At the dentist, especially, they figure the less they say without opening the mouth the better. Smart, huh. Slowly, but with a constant watch, the dentist continues tilting the dental chair back slowly into the supine position (almost flat, but not quite).

CHILD: (minding her own business) "Hi, hii, hiii," the sobbing continues, slightly low-keyed now.

DADDY: "Honey, dear, don't cry, daddy is here." As if the poor child is listening! And as if the child could forget that daddy IS indeed here, with him towering high and mighty over her.

CHILD: "Aaaii. Aaaiii, the child continues this time in the crescendo, even though the dentist is now gathering his wits and is not doing anything in the meanwhile. His hands have been withdrawn from the vicinity of her mouth for about a minute now, and is just sitting in anguish, just watching the child and watching for her to calm down a little.

DADDY: "Honey, be a good girl. This doesn't hurt at all; it won't hurt a bit; it's only like a mosquito bite."

CHILD: "AAAAAiiiii, HHHiii, AAAooo." And now the hands come up and the little trap of a mouth that actually did not offer much room to begin with is now permanently shut and sealed with all ten fingers! Little streams of tears have already cut their merry (or sorry?) path right down into each ear and now a spherical pool of water is sitting shakingly inside each little receptacle of the lower ear lobes like dew on a petal in early morning. The poor dentist is usually helpless under these situations because he cannot have a word in edgewise; the contest is now between dad and Mary!

DADDY: Don't be afraid. Remember, you promised you'll be good for Dr. T.F. (Tooth Fairy) Bruce! It won't hurt a bit.

CHILD: (Shaking her head from side to side). "I wanna go hO-O-ome, dad-d-dy, I wanna goo hoooome!" She really doesn't care what she said or promised earlier. She is taking the fifth amendment. Sue me, she is thinking.

Scenes like this, although are not very prevalent, appear to be and are all you remember when you are a dentist who sees a lot of children in a family setting. It gets so when you see a child walk into the reception area with the parent in tow you wonder what's coming next and your mood almost automatically changes. If you are not very philosophical about life you gradually become 'paedophobic' (scared of children). It is tough on the dentist just as it is tough on both the child and the parent. But parents do not have to put themselves through all this agony if only they will let the dentist do his or her thing.

Some parents, as a rule, should never be allowed into the operatory, period, for the unsettling effect they have directly on the child in the chair. Some mothers screw up their faces in such grotesque expression of disgust while the dentist is freezing the child's tooth with the needle or is cleaning a cavity with the drill that a child catching a momentary glimpse of the mother's face starts crying as if on cue. I have noticed many parents, both fathers and mothers who, although come into the treatment room ostensibly to reassure and en-COURAGE the child, would make some inaudible excuses and leave the room just as the dentist starts loading the syringe (needle) for the injection. I have seen PARENTS turn ashen white themselves, some have felt nauseous, and those who have felt faint, all because they followed their child into the operatory and then do not have the guts to stay and see it through. So, if you are that squeamish about dental work why come into the room in the first place? Parents should trust enough to leave their ward with the dental surgeon and the assistant and let them do their job the best way they know how without any interference.

There are so many ways parents can ease themselves out of the commitment to accompany a child into the treatment room even when the child wants you to. I am not a psychiatrist, but if an average, healthy six-year old child cannot undergo such simple dental procedures as an examination and a cleaning without a parent tagging along there is something lacking in the relationship — like over-protective parents? Over the years, I have observed that the children who are allowed to go for their treatment by themselves, just seem more together and are more cooperative. In fact, most of the time you already know that you are in for a difficult session when there is a fight in the reception room between the child and the parent when it is time for the child's work and the assistant goes to bring the child into the operatory.

Of course there are some children who are better patients when there is a parent around to reassure them but in my experience, this has been the exception rather than the rule. And then, from toddlers up to the age of about three years, I feel a parent needs to be there with the child anyway. As a rule, I would ask a parent into the operatory sometimes with three to five-year olds who may appear a little skittish or slightly unsure of their surroundings. But in my experience, I have found most three year-olds and upwards to be quite capable of going through a simple dental examination by themselves without any fuss.

However, the astute dentist would not hesitate to ask parents into the treatment room IF he was convinced their presence would provide a calming effect on an otherwise uncontrollable child. However, I never did and do not ever intend, asking a parent out who waltzes into the operatory in tow with the child without my summoning her. It may be against my better judgment but it is their child and I do not want any acrimonious bantering in my office. It is just a matter of courtesy on my part. I fully respect a parent's right to go anywhere their child happens to be. But under such circumstances I do not harbor any lingering sentiments of inadequacy if I was not able to bring a session to its successful completion with a parent present.

Because dentists are essentially 'surgeons' and have therefore been trained to do something other than examine, diagnose and prescribe, they tend to feel inadequate and frustrated if each treatment is not completed the way they know how and if, as in the case of a child, it happens to be on account of behavior management problems. But if the parents insist on entering the scene, it is as if they are saying to the dentist: "I know better how to deal with my child so I am here to help you out since you do not know how to handle my child." There lies my feeling exonerated; may be it is rationalization on my part but if in the presence of the parents I am still unable to behaviourally manage the child patient to do what I expect to accomplish, then I cannot be faulted for that.

The 'Greeting' After The Child's Treatment

Most dentists would rather like to do their work without the interference and the invigilation of parents. It is only after the work on the child is completed that the parent should be summoned to discuss what has been done and what else may need to be done.

Sometimes I wonder if parents come into the treatment room out of distrust or out of curiosity as to how the dentist works. But this is not a peep-show and it does more harm than good. A more prudent way to find out how the dentist works is to wait for the child in the reception area until the work is done and then ask the child about the experience.

And don't start the welcoming 'interview' with, "Honey, did it hurt?"

That insensitivity always annoyed me because it only reinforces the child's fears that it should have hurt or that mommy expected the procedure to have hurt so she cannot deny the mother her satisfaction and say it did not hurt. Depending on the child's relationship with that parent, the child may in fact answer in the positive even when in reality everything went on smoothly, not wanting to counteract mother.

The thing to do is to welcome the child with something like (and this is not the only way. This is just an example and you can find your own individual style of greeting)": Hi, Mary, you are all finished? That is good. Let me see your new filling, or let me see your nice teeth Dr. T.F. Bruce just polished for you. It's beautiful," or something to that effect. I have seen a child come out of the treatment room all smiles and then all of a sudden break out in tears just as soon as she got into the reception area and mom asked, "Did it hurt?" This is no time for sympathy. To sympathize indicates there is something noxious or unfortunate to sympathize about.

Until the child tells you it hurt, you have no business imputing your own fears on this individual who is chatting her own course and may find the experience quite different and probably more enjoyable from yours. Unless you want to prove to the child that you are always right.

CHAPTER 4

DIET, NUTRITION AND CAVITIES

In this book any reference to 'diet' simply stands for the food and drink items that one takes into the mouth. Nutrition, however, although includes what one takes into the mouth, has a more extensive meaning, like what happens to the foods you take in, its digestion, the absorption and the assimilation of the ingested food items.

It is well known in nutritional circles that protein-calorie deficiency during tooth formation can substantially increase an individual's caries susceptibility or predisposition to getting cavities. This deficiency results in 'higher than normal' susceptibility to cavities with diets that promote tooth decay. Susceptibility to tooth decay implies one naturally has a certain biologic constitution which can be influenced or affected by other environmental factors (like sugars). Whether this acquired inherent property is stronger (immunity) or weaker (susceptibility) compared to the attacking environmental factor is a question that needs answering hopefully with future research.

Here though are some facts. Sugary foods indeed do cause 'cavities'. It makes sense therefore to state that if tooth decay is accelerated by the presence of sugars in the mouth, then cavities should be inhibited if sugars are not present in the mouth. Research has systemically shown that there is a greater prevalence of cavities in children who indulge in high sugar-diets than in those with low-sugar diets.

Sugar Consumption And Cavities

Previously, when we said sugar is bad for your teeth, we generally used to refer to the variety called "SUCROSE," the most common variety of sugar consumed by humans. Sugar (i.e. sucrose) is probably not the only food item that leads to cavities but it is by far the most potent. Starches, which are complex sugars and are made up of numerous chains of many sugar units, can be broken down in the mouth into their simple sugar entities. The recommendation therefore emphasizes consumption of more UN-refined carbohydrates (e.g. potatoes, fruits, and rice). Recent studies, however, have shown that most foods containing any type of carbohydrates, monosaccharide, disaccharides, polysaccharides and even complex carbohydrates like starchy foods, can be potential causes of tooth decay.

Synergistic Effect Of Sugary Diet And Plaque Accumulation

What seems to be lost in all these discussions is the effect of multiple caries-producing factors when they appear in combination. It has been shown that the effect of persistent plaque accumulation in combination with a diet of sugary substances have a synergistic multiplicative relationship. That means the two produce an effect greater than would be expected of any one of these factors. Whilst each of these factors will certainly contribute to tooth decay, the effect is less with any one of these than the two in combination. Hence an individual who brushes routinely but feeds off sugary diet constantly may get cavities but probably less so than the one who does not brush often and consumes the same amount of sugary or acid–rich foods. There is therefore, an excess risk when these two factors are existent in the same individual.

Hence:

i. gunk (debris) on teeth + sugary foods/drinks = increased (high risk) cavity status;

ii. gunk on teeth + no sugary foods/drinks = low risk cavity status;

ii. cleaned teeth + sugary foods/drinks = moderate risk cavity status;

iv. cleaned teeth + no sugary foods/drinks = hurray...no cavity!

It is hence inappropriate to consider the effects of plaque and sugar as independent. The amount of cavities caused by plaque accumulation depends on how many of those individuals with poor oral hygiene are also exposed to frequent and increased total sugar consumption. It also means that when oral hygiene is poor, even a relatively low total sugar consumption can promote decay in those caries susceptible teeth. Researchers are baffled when they see children in rural African communities with plaque on their teeth, but are caries-free. One reason might be that the consumption of frequent sugary diets is almost negligible in these societies (ii above). Moreover, most of the carbohydrates in these African countries are in the form of complex starches or are fibrous, natural organic foods which have low cariogenic index (cause fewer cavities) compared to the simple sugary foods.

Sugar causes cavities because the causative germ, bugs or the bacteria-containing plaque, notably the MUTANS STREPTOCOCCI and the LACTOBACILLI bacteria, readily metabolize these sugars to produce : 1. Acids, and 2. Sticky products, which increase the retentiveness of the bugs and the plaque on the tooth surface. Because the bugs thrive best in acidic environments, they continue to multiply and grow as the acid production from sugar consumption continues in the mouth. The sticky substances produced by those germs as they feed on sugar also help them adhere firmly to the tooth surface and in the crevices or 'pits and fissures' especially on the back molar teeth surfaces. Cavities are therefore initiated on the smooth tooth surface as well as in the pits and fissures.

Caries Potential Of A Variety Of Foods

It used to be taught that certain food substances were more cariogenic (cavity causing) than others. It appears now that most food substances have the potential of causing tooth decay as long as they stay in the mouth long enough to be used by the sugar-bugs in the mouth and acids produced from them. Foods that before used to be thought of as 'good' against cavities e.g. apples, and carrots, have all been found to in fact possess fermentable sugars (could cause tooth decay) if left in the mouth long enough, like more than 24 hours without cleaning. If the food is retentive and therefore stays in the mouth longer, it can be used by the bugs or bacteria with resultant acid production. The longer the food stays on the teeth, the more potential it has to form acids and therefore promotes tooth decay.

Fruit Juices And Cavities

Fermentable sugars, i.e. sugars that can be used by sugar-bugs to produce acids, e.g. glucose, fructose and sucrose and many organic acids are ubiquitous in fruits. In ripe fruits, the predominant free acids are: **malic acid (as in apples, apricots, bananas, cherries, and grapes), citric acid (in lemons, oranges currants, figs, gooseberries, guava, pomegranates, raspberries and strawberries) and tartaric acid (as in grapes).** These and many other weak acids, in association with potassium, constitute acid juices with strong buffering systems. Vitamin C, which occurs naturally in most fresh fruits, contributes to some of the acidity in fruit juices. Saliva, thank God for the lowly-regarded 'spit', slowly neutralizes dietary acids, thereby minimizing or controlling the initiation of tooth decay. Although saliva is well endowed with a strong naturally buffering or neutralizing system, it no longer is effective when the critical acidity of the oral environment (or the pH at which tooth enamel dissolves) reaches 5.0 to 5.5; the problem is that most fruit juices have a pH well below this critical point. Remember, the lower the pH, the more the acidity, and the faster the tooth substance is demineralized (softens tooth structure) into forming a cavity.

Parents and patients alike should be aware of the damage fruit juices can do to the teeth. Increased consumption of fruit juices frequently makes teeth sensitive. The high acidity juice softens the tooth structure by dissolving the calcium in the outer tooth enamel. Patients should therefore be advised against sucking frozen juice and drinking juices before bed. Children should also not be regularly fed fruit juices in feeding bottles, or in frozen cubes for extended periods of time.

Strategies to minimize the dental effects of fruit juices are:
1. drinking juices through a straw;
2. diluting the juice with water;
3. rinsing mouth with water after drinking juice;
4. reducing frequency of drinking juices;
5. consuming it as part of a meal and not as an isolated snack.

Rinsing the mouth with an alkaline mouthwash or toothpaste after an acid drink is advisable. Because it is felt that brushing the teeth immediately after a fruit juice drink is not advisable, as softened tooth enamel may be abraded by brushing, it is probably better to instead rinse the mouth with a mouthwash or even with water soon after (as in 3 above).

But even this statement needs qualification. YOU CAN INDEED EAT YOUR CAKE AND STILL KEEP YOUR TEETH. In fact, you can eat your usual dose of sweets and acidic foods and juices and still be caries-free depending upon WHEN you eat these and WHAT you do after eating them.

To be free of 'cavities', sticky, gummy foods (yes, like bread, cookies, potato chips) are a no-no if you cannot brush or rinse after you've had them. These adhere to the teeth for long periods of time and are therefore more available to the sugar-bugs for production of the acids which then attack the teeth. How often you eat these is also a factor. If you ate these foods all day, especially in between meals you will be courting BIIIG trouble. However, if you eat these at meal times, you'll be home free, particularly if you brush or rinse your teeth afterwards. Even rinsing the mouth after a meal with copious amounts of water or chewing sugarless gum is enough to help clear some of the acid-producing food particles out of the mouth, this eliminating the possibility of you being the constant provider for your not-so-friendly sugar-bugs. One particularly sugarless gum, those with xylitol as the sugar substitute, aside of producing copious amounts of saliva in the mouth because of the chewing action and thus helping to neutralize acids produced by the bugs, have also been found to actually arrest (stop) further development of small, incipient (beginning) 'cavities.'

Chewing on a piece of cheese, meat or nuts, thereby producing copious amounts of saliva which will help neutralize the acids produced in the mouth after the meal, is also recommended.

I used to think (and hey, did I want to believe!) that eating chocolate bars with nuts (like nutchos and other such delicious favourites) is a sweet way to kill two birds with one stone. You get to satisfy your sweet tooth and not have to worry about getting 'cavities' because of the presence of the nuts. A study done at the University of Ghana Dental School, with dark, Ghanaian chocolate, has in fact collaborated my belief – that the nuts in these chocolates indeed reduce acidity in the mouth and therefore will not promote cavities. But note—it should be the dark chocolate variety, not the regular reformulated mixed chocolates.

Saliva— Or — Spit — And Dry Mouth

"Spit" may be a dirty word but it helps clean your mouth like you wouldn't believe. Saliva or spit, together with all the other good things it does for us humans, helps neutralize the acids produced after meals as has already been mentioned. Nature's conditioning, where we start salivating when we smell food cooking (which Pavlov so very clearly elucidated in his experiments with his dog), is a way we are naturally prepared and readied to protect our teeth as well as helping to digest the foods we eat.

But the production and protection of saliva in the mouth decreases as we age, making us more susceptible to tooth decay. People with dry mouth or **xerostomia** where saliva production is reduced either because of disease, medication or just mere old age, therefore, have to see their dentist to replace the now non-existent, naturally-produced saliva with artificial saliva preparations.

CHAPTER 5

DENTAL DISEASE – THE THREE MAIN TYPES

There are three major categories of dental diseases that a dentist is called upon to treat. These are: cavities, gum diseases and general diseases of the mouth.

5A. Tooth Decay— "Cavities"

These are the well-known 'holes' that appear on and inside the teeth. Cavities, decay, 'caries' (this word is only used in the plural), or 'carious lesions,' describe the same phenomenon and are used by dentists interchangeably.

But a tooth decay, a 'carious lesion' or a cavity does not have to be a hole. In fact, in the average individual, unless they have been neglected for years, a carious lesion shows for the most part, and initially, at least, not as a definite hole but a hidden internal softening of the tooth structure only evident to the trained eye or on an x-ray. Hence the reluctance of dentists to use the everyday term of a 'cavity' and the preference for the term 'decay', 'caries' or 'a carious lesion' which accurately and scientifically describes the disease state. The preference for the right choice of terminology is to impress on the general public that even though there may not be a definite hole in the tooth that there still could be a 'cavity' present. If dentists routinely demonstrated to their patients the presence of a lesion on the x-ray may be there would not be the wrongful suspicion that some "dentist has filled teeth even though there were no holes anywhere on them". What I find disturbing is the patient who comes in and says—" doctor, I have a chipped tooth". These individuals, in an attempt to get away from the admission and therefore self- incrimination that they have an infection in their tooth, would use the euphemism of a 'chip' for a cavity. You cannot deceive the dentist especially when the 'chip' has been there for a year or so, has gotten bigger and is now bothering you when food gets in.

I have also heard patients accuse dentists of filling the wrong teeth. This situation usually occurs mainly because the patient describes the experienced toothache as emanating from a certain part of the mouth. The dentist examines the area and finds a decayed, bad tooth on the x-ray and proceeds to restore (fill) this tooth. Because the ache does not go away right after the filling, it is automatically assumed that he filled the wrong tooth. And then in some cases the tooth the patient felt was the culprit may not in fact have any decay on it. But the only way to dispel all suspicion and misunderstanding is for the dentist to first (1) show and explain clearly to the patient that these are his findings and (2) obtain the patient's consent to fix the tooth he feels needs attention.

What Is a Cavity?

The diagnosis of a 'cavity" when it is in its very small or initial (incipient) developmental stages is an area of great debate in dentistry. Two dentists may not count the same number of teeth with 'cavities' in the same mouth. I remember, while a graduate student in Public Health Dentistry, I was fortunate enough to be chosen as one of two examiners in a survey study to determine the extent of dental disease within a population of some institutionalized senior citizens. The other examiner was then a practicing dentist while I had been in Dental Public Health training already for about two years. Believe it or not there were some differences in our counts of dental decay on many of the people examined. As a rule, what one dentist would call a 'cavity' may not be so designated by another dentist. Public Health Dentists may not call it a 'cavity', because of their special training in population studies, what some practicing dentists would so designate. And to complicate it further, because of the non-uniformity of dental education in Universities, different schools teach the students different rationales for detecting carious lesions. Moreover, some unscrupulous dentists, I hear, would fill every small cavity they see—even those they could wait and watch— for economic reasons—to make more money.

Hence, in my practice, I would stress this point to patients that there are teeth that may or may not be deemed to have 'cavities'. There may in fact be an indication of a cavity in a particular tooth but the lesion may be so small that it may not be worth 'chasing' after and destroying good tooth structure. This we put on 'watch' or on observation at subsequent visits to ensure they do not get worse. Of course you have a problem if the patient stops coming for frequent check-ups. But then they had been apprised already of the presence of these small lesions so you hope they will comply and continue their regular visits, even if it is in another clinic.

Why Do We Get 'Cavities'

Part Played By Heredity

As a dental student, I was taught that we get 'cavities' from eating sugary foods and from not brushing our teeth properly. In spite of that, and from many observations, I am still convinced that although sugar may present part of the answer that heredity plays a big part in the causation of 'carious lesions.' In my practice, I have had to rationalize why children from the same family eating approximately the same types of foods exhibit such diverse susceptibilities (inherent propensities) to developing 'cavities.' Moreover, we are all aware of siblings, one of whom brushes religiously and still develops a lot of 'cavities' while the other who does not even own a toothbrush is free of 'cavities.'

I still feel very strongly that the inherent propensity to develop 'cavities' is inherited and this susceptibility is played out by the superimposition of environmental factors like fluorides and poor habits like frequent ingestion of sugar-containing foods and/or improper home care techniques. Moreover, it is now known that siblings with varying levels of decay do not differ in the type of carbohydrates eaten but rather the differing amounts and frequency with which each respectively indulged in the eating habit.

The attack rate of tooth decay is a chance (probability) phenomenon which I feel depends on how strong the inherent abilities or inabilities to resist tooth decay and prevent its development are in the individual. Hence, I believe that caries susceptibility (or resistance) is a characteristic or property of the tooth substance itself. Some dental experts argue that although the pattern of tooth decay in individuals may indicate some genetic influence, that environmental factors (like sugars) have greater influence. So be it, but either way that means genetics play some part, however small.

The part played by heredity in conferring susceptibility to dental disease has not been thoroughly studied although resistance to disease has been found in a few instances to be a function of genes, and in a majority of cases several genes appear to be involved.

Another reason for my own strong belief in the power of the underlying inheritance of risk to forming 'cavities' is the fact that the mere possession, even of high amounts, of the bacteria reputed to be the culprit in the development of caries – mutans Streptococci— is not necessarily sufficient to make one cavity-prone. When I was an undergraduate dental student, my class studied this phenomenon. Of the twenty-two odd students, I ranked the second highest in the possession of the Strep. mutans, the putative "cavity" bacteria. And yet, I had the least amount of fillings (only 3) and with only one decayed tooth to my name. The other two fillings I already had were two contiguous teeth I fractured at one of our dental school parties when I was gleefully opening beer bottles with my teeth. Some dental student! Huh! This Strep. mutans test was illogical and very insensitive (not identifying those who actually are cavity-prone) unless there are other factors still to be identified; moreover, I was not one for sugarless foods; I ate my share of chocolate bars and ice creams like any other average Canadian citizen. Sure, I brushed often enough, but was that enough to infer a near zero cavity rate on a twenty-six year old student? This idea of resistance or immunity to decay in some people has not been studied thoroughly yet but must play a big part in the caries experience of individuals.

Another example is found in many parts of Africa. Almost all studies coming out of Africa indicate that generally the people have far less decayed teeth than in their respective age groups in developed countries. And yet, most of these African countries do not have half the dental care amenities prevalent in the Western countries — like water fluoridation, fluoridated toothpastes, fluoride rinses and the like. To compound it all, the staple dishes in many African countries are loaded with carbohydrates, but generally of the complex starchy types. With high amounts of the mutans Streptococci in the presence of slowly-cleansed complex carbohydrates, this population should be inundated with tooth decay. But they are not. Does this not, quoting Arsenio Hall's famous saying, make you say, "Hmmm?"

One of my Lecturers in my undergrad days always insisted that if the African were to be challenged with nutrition as in North America that they would succumb to high prevalence of caries. Although this has not been tested unequivocally yet the high influx of immigrants and refugees into Canada these days has given us some partial answers to this question. It has been noticed that although these refugees would come in with lower caries prevalence that they experience a higher susceptibility after a few years of stay in Canada. The susceptibility changes as a result of different environmental exposures into a high risk status. So I guess my Prof was right, huh.

Now here is the rub. How does one know a child is at risk for tooth decay? The problem is that risk to dental diseases can, so far as our knowledge goes, be assessed retrospectively and ONLY after the fact or a posteriori, in the sense that it is only after the child has experienced the disease that a risk can be imputed. Research is still going on and in the very near future such risk assessment techniques will be available where an individual can be determined to be at risk for dental disease and can then assume the primary preventive orientation before any disease is experienced.

It is at this point that my belief in heredity comes in. At the present, the only way to assess how your child is going to fare in this elusive dental disease experience is through the property of the 'quality' of the tooth structure. Since it is true that we inherit the morphology (the shape, form and size of teeth) as well as the bone structure of the jaws, why should the "quality" be different? In any case if both parents have a very low susceptibility to tooth decay it is very probable that the children will also experience very low caries rates. If both parents have high disease experience then it is very probable that the children will demonstrate the same susceptibility, due, also in part, to the interplay of environmental factors. Where one parent has high caries experience but the other does not, the children may probably show mixed rates. But then it may also be that as the saying goes in West Africa, 'a crab does not beget a bird' or to put it in another way, 'like mother like daughter.' If the parents don't take good care for their own teeth, they probably do not take good care of their children's teeth either and hence the similarities in their tooth decay experience.

Immunity Or Resistance To Dental Disease

With all said and done, even immunity or resistance to dental disease is a difficult phenomenon to ascribe to anyone unless the individual has been challenged first and has not shown any susceptibility. This is because the extent to which an individual may be susceptible or resistant is determined by the interaction of many factors. It is therefore possible that your child may well appear to be 'immune' to tooth decay but may contract the disease later on through environmental influences. It is believed that persons are susceptible to a disease when, upon exposure to the necessary conditions, that they will contract the affliction because their biology, physiology (how the body functions), and even their psychology and lifestyle make them responsive. In one research publication, the only state where anyone is defined as being anything close to being immune or resistant to tooth decay is where "the individual is 17 years or over, who has never had any decay, restored (filled) or extracted (pulled) teeth (except wisdom teeth or through an accident) although has been exposed to normal environmental challenge". You see how difficult it is therefore to say at the onset that a child is resistant to tooth decay? If the definition says 17 years or over, till what age? At what age, therefore, can one then say, OK now, I am really immune to tooth decay? And, what is "normal environmental challenge?" Isn't it normal in the conditions under which this individual already finds him/herself?

5B. Preventive Dentistry In Children

When we talk of primary prevention, we mean techniques used to prevent dental diseases BEFORE they attack. This is differentiated from what has classically been termed 'secondary prevention' which deals with detecting any disease AFTER the attack by, hopefully, catching it at its very early stages. At this point, the disease is already present but at its very incipient (early) stage.

As discussed (in Chapter 3), taking care of the baby's mouth before and after the eruption of the teeth is the first stage in the primary preventive process. Other methods applied to ensure a caries-free mouth will be discussed here.

A child's dental care should be started as soon as he or she is born. This is because babies are not born with a mouth full of cavity-causing bacteria. It is felt that babies acquire these bacteria from the parents through such loving activities as feeding procedures, cuddling, hugging and kissing. The bacterial colonization in a child's mouth does not happen in an instant, but is acquired repeatedly, a little at a time. This is why some dental authorities feel tooth decay is an "infectious disease". Nursing mothers, nurturing fathers and even grandmothers should therefore take care of their own mouths in order to ensure a healthy state for the baby. This is done by brushing or cleaning your own mouth at least twice a day (preferably with a fluoridated toothpaste), flossing regularly and keeping at least one yearly appointments (or whatever time interval is appropriate or appeals to you) with your dentist.

Wiping the baby's gums after feeding with a wet cloth, a clean towel or face cloth will do. When the new teeth start popping into the mouth, keep this cleaning schedule up. You can now even add a very small amount of fluoridated toothpaste (pea-size) on the towel to clean the teeth.

We used to think that a child who is breast-fed will not develop cavities from the mother's milk but we now know that there is no difference between the breast and the feeding bottle in so far as sugar-bugs are concerned. These bugs don't discriminate just because it is now the breast supplying the food. Breast milk is therefore just as easily fermented as the milk from the bottle, and they can both cause tooth decay if used as "pacifiers." It is a wonder that children in many African countries don't have a mouthful of cavities. In many of these regions, the breast is a typical pacifier (only for the kids, you dirty old man!) and is at the beck and call of the baby. The slightest whimper from the child and the tired mother rolls one of these heavy, papaya-sized, drooping, milk-engorged bazookas from in front and directs it backward or sideways towards the child who is in the meanwhile strapped on the mother's back. It is surprising, because in the African society where breast-feeding is a very common practice and is done by mothers in the market place and everywhere, as long as the kid wants it, one would expect the kids to have mouths full of holes, and yet they are not. And the interesting observation is that most of the kids are weaned very late from breast-feeding. Is it possible that African mothers have adequate fluoride in their breast-milk? Or that their breast milk contains other caries fighting minerals from their consumption of the ubiquitous well water? It is known, for example, that in Northern Ghana that most of the wells contain so much fluoride that there is a big problem with fluorosis.

Fluorides

Fluoride, in many different forms, is still the main vehicle presently known in dentistry to be the most effective agent against tooth decay.

Water fluoridation has been known to be associated with less tooth decay in children for years. Also, it has been shown over and over again that adults who are born, raised and continue to live in a fluoridated community demonstrate markedly better dental health than do adults in non-fluoridated communities. Hence, fluoridation of communal water supplies should be the cornerstone upon which any national program of dental caries prevention is built. "Fluoridation constitutes nearly an ideal public health program in that benefits are conferred regardless of family socio-economic level, education or the availability of dental manpower." It appears that in developed countries, even those regions with no community fluoridated water systems still get the benefit because of the 'halo effect.' That means even those areas not directly drinking the fluoridated water are indirectly exposed to some immeasurable amounts of fluoride through public consumption of variously available foods and beverages manufactured with fluoridated water from far away factories.

Prenatal Fluoride Intake

This is a very contentious area of discussion, but the dental community generally believes that no good rationale exists for mothers to take prenatal fluoride supplements. In moderate amounts it may not hurt the mother any but it is probably not necessary. Where there is the optimum fluoride content in the drinking water there appears no need for the mother or child to take fluoride supplements. Supplements may, however, be necessary if the community water supply is not fluoridated and the children happen to be at risk for tooth decay.

Different Forms Of Fluorides And Tooth Resistance

From above discussions, it is evident that where in doubt it may be prudent to cover your child with fluoride supplements even when there is fluoride in the community water to start with. Your dentist will be able to prescribe a suitable and appropriate fluoride medium for your child, depending upon the age. If you live in a rural area or on a farm and you have your own water system you may want to have it tested for its fluoride content first to determine if supplements will be needed. But it is suggested that if needed, supplements should be started at an age not earlier than six months.

Fluoride can also be given in the form of a topical gel or varnish applications right on the teeth to strengthen them. Or the gel may be placed in a foam tray and inserted over the teeth and left to sit anywhere from one to four minutes. It is recommended that after the application of the topical fluoride that the child does not eat or drink for at least thirty minutes. This allows the tooth enamel more time to take in the fluoride to form a more resistant layer, which layer of enamel, then, helps resist the effects of acid produced by the ever-present sugar bugs in the mouth.

It is also recommended to have this application done twice in the year (or once every six months) for a significant effect.

Fluoride topical gels or varnishes are to be used in selected individuals determined to be at risk for increased tooth decay. This means not everybody should have this fluoride treatment. Because of its high fluoride concentration it is to be used either in the dental office or by a trained individual so that proper supervision can be given.

Toothpastes

The same beneficial fluoride effect is obtained from the use of fluoride-containing toothpastes. There are nowadays all kinds of these on the market with all forms of fluoride formulations and other additives to enhance the effect of the fluoride (1000-1200 ppm fl). As long as the tooth paste contains adequate amounts of fluoride, you should only choose these on the basis of your taste and perhaps the level of abrasiveness desired, especially if you are a smoker. And be prepared to brush for at least three to five minutes both to do a good enough cleaning job and also to allow more time for the fluoride to be absorbed onto your teeth surfaces.

Fluoride Rinses

Your child may come home and report that there is a fluoride rinse program in the school. This is usually provided in a group setting since it is more cost effective. However, if desired, your dentist will prescribe a type for your use at home. However, fluoride rinses should be prescribed only to children over six years old who have developed the ability to rinse and only to those who have been shown to be at risk. There are rinses for daily as well as weekly use for children. The fluoride mouth rinse should, however, not be used as a substitute for the more effective topical gel application. The rinse can be added as an adjunct to fight the general onslaught of tooth decay.

So You Have A 'Cavity' – How Is It Fixed?

Fillings

Most decayed teeth are filled with regular filling materials. To the dentist a filling is not just a 'filling.' Hence asking for the price of a 'filling' is not totally meaningful. Each tooth has five surfaces exposed in the mouth, any or all these surfaces can decay and so the 'filling' may involve anywhere from one to five surfaces and thus deserving of specific fee. Some dentists would charge a multiple of the fee for one surface if the cavities involve more than one surface. Generally, however, the fee guide is designed to charge incrementally as the number of surfaces increased.

These days because of the debate on the merits or demerits of the gray metal filling (the traditional 'amalgam' or 'silver' filling), a white filling may be used to fill even the back teeth. There is no question as to what dentists traditionally have and would continue to use to fill a front tooth. The front teeth have always been filled with white filings which may be 'acrylic', filled acrylic or 'composite' material, or porcelain. Some cultures used to prefer gold for the front teeth as a sign of 'having arrived' or to show one's elevated social status but this practice is not as popular as it used to be.

Nowadays one has the choice to have the back teeth filled with white composite or porcelain material instead of the gray 'silver' or amalgam filling. These attract higher fees than the 'silver' fillings because of the high research and manufacturing costs and the more involved techniques encountered in their utilization at the dentist's office.

It should be mentioned here that just because a tooth has been 'filled' does not mean that all future work on it is completed and that nothing can go wrong with it ever again. All filling materials used presently, with the exception of cast gold fillings (more on these materials later), can fracture with use. Hence a 'silver' or white composite filling can crack or fracture and may need to be replaced.

If, because of procrastination or mere neglect, a 'cavity' was deep to begin with, filling such a tooth is not necessarily the end of it. The dentist cleans the tooth by removing all obvious decay until in his judgment all the 'carious lesion' is removed. I said "in his judgement" because in fact this process of cleaning the cavity, in theory and in most practical cases, may not completely remove all the decay. Chasing after the decay even when the tooth is to all intents and purposes 'clean', however, only gets one dangerously close to the tooth pulp (the 'nerve'). In such cases, a dressing 'filling' (a lining or a base) is placed over the deepest aspect of the cleaned 'cavity' before the second layer of filling is packed on top of the dressing. A tooth treated this way may never bother the individual again or may start aching as early as the following week, the next month or the following year. It probably depends on so many factors like reduced body resistance at certain periods in one's life, the extent of the encroachment into the pulp (nerve) area or the amount and manner of use of the particular tooth. But for whatever reason or reasons some filled teeth can act up again and the time factor is anyone's guess. Baring fracture, and this is just an experiential calculation, a filling should last for at least five to seven years.

This problem of fracture applies to both adult 'permanent' and baby ('deciduous') teeth although it may be seen more in baby teeth. This is because the baby teeth have bigger pulp area ('nerve') compared to the tooth size and the decay generally progresses a lot faster than in adult teeth.

Sealants

Thanks for the availability of acrylic 'flowable' fillings, a susceptible tooth surface can now be 'sealed off' such that tooth bugs cannot get to it to start a cavity. As you can easily verify in the mirror, all molar teeth, the big chewing teeth at the back, have grooves on them. These grooves as a result of the natural process of tooth formation present a rough surface for more efficient chewing. Otherwise, a tooth surface will be very smooth and one will not be able to chew that effectively. The problem is that the same grooves on the top surfaces of the chewing teeth are also the very sites where the tooth bugs love to reside comfortably unmolested by your toothbrush, and multiply undisturbed. In some people the grooves are very deep and can trap food and plaque within them, facilitating the onset of tooth decay. These individuals belong to the group of people who will particularly benefit from the application of sealants on their molar teeth surfaces.

Sealants of acrylic material and in flow-able form initially, are applied to the top surfaces of these molar teeth where the sealant material flows into the crevices of the grooves. The flow-able liquid sealant is then hardened with 'a hardening flash-light' and helps seal the grooves off from the invasion of the tooth bugs.

Sealants are therefore of more benefit if used on children just as these molar teeth are erupting into the mouth. It is more efficient if applied within the first two years of a tooth's eruption, since the tooth's susceptibility to decay decreases with time. Hence sealants are indicated mostly for the ages of six to eight years, (for the first permanent molars) and 13 to 15 years (for the second permanent molars). It is therefore almost a waste of time and money if a tooth is sealed four or five years after its eruption into the mouth. If the chewing surface of a back tooth has not decayed within three to four years of its eruption it is not susceptible enough to merit a sealant since it would now have passed its maturation ("hardening") stage.

5C. Gum Disease

The Canadian Dental Association Awareness Program Report published in 1985 was replete with a pressing message both to the dental professionals and the public at large:

"More than four-fifths of Canadians expect to lose their teeth. Nearly a quarter of the population, only see a dentist for specific problems. They see no threat from periodontal disease. In short, although they might want to prevent dental disease, they don't expect to be successful and they don't know how to do it;

Canadians are sadly ignorant about periodontal disease. Not only is ignorance widespread, but regular patients are just as confused as the general population. This indicates a serious failure to communicate effectively with Canadians about periodontal disease. Dentists bear considerable responsibility for these problems, and they must take the initiative to solve it." Although, this statement was made back in 1985, there is no indication that conditions have changed much.

Gum Disease, Still The Most Misunderstood

Of all dental diseases, I feel the second most misunderstood and misrepresented is GUM DISEASE (root canal treatment takes the first place). It is so insidious and as it were, 'comes as a thief in the night' that many people have found individualized reasons to explain away why their teeth have loosened. It appears there must have been a rash of accidents approximately 30 years ago because in most cases where I have diagnosed teeth that are loose I have gotten such unique answers as: "I had a car accident when I was young", "I was hit in the mouth at work by a jack" or the other favourite, "I was kicked in the mouth by a horse." And these people are in their late forties or fifties! These teeth have been accidentally loosened thirty years ago and have just decided to loosen up now, tell me another one! Those in their thirties often ascribe loosened teeth to playing hockey.

People generally hate to be told bluntly that it is because they have not been brushing well or are just not 'taking care of their teeth and gums.' Coupled with the fact that most of these loosened teeth are in all segments (regions) of the mouth, it makes you wonder where the preferred site for these presumed accidents were. Not many people know enough or dare to connect the presence of the heavy collection of tartar around the gum-line of their teeth to the eventual loosening of these teeth. It comes as a shock in fact to many of these 'accident victims' when you draw their attention to the fact that they are losing their teeth simply because of the presence of that 'insignificant' layer of hard brown substance on the teeth. Some patients, with a straight face, actually try to convince you that this dark substance lining the teeth at the gum line is "part of their teeth chipping off." It comes therefore as a great revelation when you quietly chip off a piece of the tartar (a chip off the 'old block') to show them, revealing underneath a whole tooth and nothing but the tooth, pun definitely intended. The only answer that I usually give to their –"What caused that?" is simply "from not brushing or cleaning the teeth properly," which in 'truth' is the whole answer.

Some Definitions First— Tooth Anatomy

The next time you hear your dentist say you have a 'periodontal' disease just substitute 'gum disease' and you may be right on. Without boring you with any extensive dental anatomy let us get into just a light description of the tooth structure to demonstrate some very important points.

Each tooth consists of two parts: the CROWN, the part you see sticking out into the mouth, and the ROOT(S), the 'usually' unseen portion hidden in the jaw bone **and by the way people look incredulous when told that each tooth is sitting inside the bone?** The NECK of this tooth is therefore where the crown and the root(s) meet at the gum line. The gum ('gingiva') is the protective soft skin that clings to the necks of the teeth and covers the bone holding the teeth. Hence, 'periodontal' disease ('peri-' around, '-odont-al' of the tooth), means disease around the tooth or disease of the structures surrounding the tooth, technically the gum and the bone. Some teeth usually have two or three supporting roots. Inside, in the middle of each tooth like a straw in a bottle or the wick inside a candle, is the nerve which keeps the tooth alive.

With that out of the way, let us find out how we can take care of our teeth and gums the effective way.

Signs of Periodontal Disease

A normal healthy gum should be pink and firm around the teeth. People with darker, pigmented skins (or non-whites) have gums quite a bit darker on account of the natural presence of the pigment in the gums. Even some whites who may have had "a black connection" a long time ago in their genealogical history would exhibit some pigmentation to a varying degree. Most of the time these pigments would be evident around the gums surrounding the upper front teeth and in the gums in the palate of the top jaw.

This reminds me of my dental school days in Canada, in our third year of training, when we were being initiated into the science and the art of diagnosing gum problems. One of my mates had the misfortune of having a black girl of about fourteen years for dental examination. While discussing his findings, he diagnosed the 'funny blackish looking gums' as a sign of cancer! Of course we had taken the theoretical oral pathology course in the previous year, where we learnt about certain pigmented cancerous abnormalities in humans. It goes without saying that this diagnosis was met with guffaws and some ridicule for the uppity beginning clinician who thought he had diagnosed cancer in one of his first batch of assigned patients. But this is really not funny because dentists who have not come into contact with black patients may make similar mistakes. Never mind— patients themselves are baffled when they see such blackish pigmentation on their gums. When I used to work with Aboriginals many of the patients, mostly women, were at a loss when they found these black stains on their gums—dirty gums, they would ask—and I would answer them that it is not dirt but are black pigmentations and might very well indicate a black relationship in their ancestry way way back. Surprise surprise!

Pigmentation aside, how do you know if your gums are healthy? Do you want to keep your teeth for the rest of your life? If you do, then consider taking care of both the teeth and the surrounding gums. If your gums exhibit all or some of the symptoms discussed below see your dentist so that he can provide the appropriate treatment.

1. Red and Puffy Gums: No matter what your normal skin complexion, your gums should not appear red, puffy, swollen or shiny.

2. Bleeding Gums: Healthy gums should not bleed under normal circumstances, even when brushed or flossed, unless you are not flossing properly. If your gums bleed, even sometimes, then something is wrong and you should visit the dentist. A regular soft to medium toothbrush should not cause gum bleeding.

3. Halitosis or Persistent Bad Breadth: Bad breadth can be a sign of periodontal or gum disease. It may be difficult to notice this yourself so check with your family or intimate friends to help by telling you.

4. Receding Gums: Your gums should be positioned just around the necks of the teeth. Diseased gums in some cases will cause the gums to shrink away from the tooth crown, expose the neck and sometimes part of the root(s). This makes the teeth look longer. It may also result in the teeth being painfully sensitive around the neck region, especially to sweets, acidic foods or cold drinks.

    Some minor recession (receding gums) may not necessarily be caused by periodontal disease but may be just a part of the normal aging process or due to improper tooth-brushing method. However, any receding of the gums at any age should alert one until the dentist says it is normal for you.

5. Loosening of one or more teeth.

6. The teeth begin to drift around and show more spacing.

7. Itching, a diffuse or vague ache or other gum discomfort may be an indication that there might be a disease process going on in the gums.

What really causes Gum Disease?

Gingivitis

Everyday as you eat, a sticky, almost invisible film (biofilm) forms on the teeth. This film is called PLAQUE or BIOFILM. In large amounts plaque can be seen, particularly around the gum-line and you can actually feel the plaque as a fuzzy, slightly rough, unclean coating on the teeth.

Admixed within this sticky film are remnants of food debris as well as a growing colony of 'sugar bugs' or bacteria. We all have bugs or bacteria in our mouths. The physical presence of the plaque, plus the fact that the bugs within it are continuously feeding off the food remnants and producing poisonous by-products like acids and other toxins combine to inflame (irritate) the gums. This irritation or inflammation of the gums is called 'GINGIVITIS' and is the initial stages of gum or periodontal disease.

In its mild form gingivitis is evident when the gums begin to change colour from the normally healthy pink to a reddish colour in certain areas of the gum margins and the papillary regions (the triangular-shaped bits of gum in between the teeth). In the moderate to the severe cases the cherry-like redness is accompanied by puffiness and swelling of the gums, and bleeding when touched (as in brushing or when just eating). Bleeding can occur spontaneously as in during sleep. Those who drool may find blood on the pillow and usually will blame it on mosquito bites during the night.

Plaque Becomes Tartar

If you do not brush your teeth for about a day (from about four hours onwards) plaque will start forming on your teeth. If this plaque is not disturbed for days, it may then start forming tartar. Depending on the type of saliva you have and your predisposition, the plaque may become hardened by addition of calcium from your saliva and soon form the crusty, hard, rough substance on the teeth called tartar or 'calculus.' The physical presence of this foreign, abnormal tartar plus the fact that the bugs within it continue feeding off the food remnants and producing poisonous toxins combine to aggravate the gum inflammation (infection). Although tartar itself is hard underneath, there is always some soft plaque or bugs on top of it feeding off food debris you have left on your teeth.

Once the calculus (tartar) forms on your teeth, you cannot remove it yourself, not even with a hard toothbrush. It clings to the teeth with such tenacity that only a dental professional can remove it for you. You see it as the brownish or black deposit or discolouration around the necks of the teeth. You should, however, keep the teeth clean by removing the soft layer of plaque.

I am always amazed at how perfectly ordered nature is. Here are these infinitesimal, microscopic organisms (bacteria) and yet they are so incredibly evolved that they will form a thin layer on human teeth with such precision and tenacity that it will not peel off no matter how hard you scrub the teeth. It is a wonder to me how tenacious this tartar can get to the extent that sometimes even the machine used to remove it has a hard time of it. And yet, dentists with all the twenty-first century technology cannot even keep a lousy filling inside a tooth permanently without it fracturing or falling off! Incredible, isn't it? But that is nature for you!

There are two areas on the tooth where calculus habitually forms. It is easily seen around the gums on the teeth but then grows downward into and around the gum-line. As it grows some of it becomes embedded UNDER the gums so that you cannot often see this extension of it. It is this hidden tartar under the gums that does most harm to the gums and to the underlying bone.

All tartar will always have plaque embedded on its surface and all plaque is capable of starting or worsening periodontal (gum) disease.

The areas in the mouth most affected by calculus collection are:

1. the inside (tongue side) of the lower front teeth and

2. the outside cheek side of the top back molar teeth. This is because these particular areas are closest to saliva producing glands which therefore facilitate the calcification of plaque that forms in these regions.

Bone Loss, Pocket Formation and Pyorrhea

The toxins (poisons) produced by the bacteria ('bugs') in the plaque not only inflame (infect) the gum (gingivitis) but also cause the destruction of the bone supporting the teeth.

The root of each tooth is surrounded, supported and held firmly inside and under the gums by the jaw bone. As gum infection progresses, the destruction of the bone surrounding the tooth is initiated, with no appreciable symptoms in this early stages of the disease. As bone destruction continues, a diseased region develops around the tooth which is now filled with breakdown products of dead bacteria, toxins, bits of dead gum lining, food debris and blood products. This diseased region works its way down along the root surface within its bony envelope and soon causes the deepening of the crevice around each tooth. At this point a 'POCKET' has been formed around the tooth.

Sometimes the pocket, together with all its diseased contents, may form 'pus' which you can actually see when you press your finger against the diseased gums surrounding the tooth. It is this formation of pus from the diseased gum AND bone around the tooth which gives this stage the name of 'PYORRHOEA' or an abscess. Whenever your dentist says you have an abscess that means not only are your gums diseased but the underlying supporting bone is affected as well and there is pus in the area.

As some of you readers will attest to, the diseased contents of the gum 'pocket' can inadvertently be expressed into the mouth, explaining the bad taste. These pocket contents can also cause bad breath. But of course one can also have bad breadth from the initial 'gingivitis' stage from not brushing off the accumulated food debris and the bugs or plaque.

A periodontal (gum) disease therefore without bone loss is called 'gingivitis', meaning only the soft gums have been affected. Once the gum starts being stripped from the neck of the tooth and the underlying bone becomes involved, the stage now becomes the more serious 'periodontal disease' and teeth may start loosening (this is now periodontitis).

There is one form of periodontal disease not caused a priori by improper home care although may be aggravated by the lack of good home care. This has to do with a naturally occurring insufficient width of gum zone around the teeth. This is usually treated with a surgical lengthening of or addition to the surrounding gums to provide the optimum width needed for the more efficient protection of the teeth.

Problem With Untreated periodontal Diseases

One of the most obvious sequela (result) of periodontal disease is the loosening and loss of teeth. The other occurrence is swelling of the jaw beside the periodontally involved tooth. Bad breadth and a nasty or unpleasant taste in the mouth can also occur at any phase of a periodontal infection. Left untreated for a long time (how long is any one's guess) it can actually affect the tooth itself and lead to the 'death' and an eventual loss of the tooth in the form of dental abscess where the pulp ('nerve') of the tooth becomes infected. A lot of periodontitis goes unnoticed because in the very chronic forms the gums may look very normal, pink, hard but bulbous, with no bleeding. The only indication might be some 'itchy' or funny feeling in the gums. The thing to do if you want to know is to visit your neighbourhood dentist, like a year ago?

If you notice these problems in your mouth you most probably have gum or periodontal disease:
  a. red, tender (sore), inflamed (bulbous, enlarged) gums;
  b. bleeding gums while brushing, flossing or even eating;
  c. bad breath, odour;
  d. Loose or loosening teeth' shifting of the teeth or gradual increased spacing of the teeth.

It surprises me how people who pride themselves as clean and neat live constantly with dirty mouths and don't think much of it. To me the mouth is a very sensitive indicator of good breeding and cleanliness. And I don't mean nice crowns and gold work and implants. I mean just simple cleaning the teeth and mouth AT LEAST once a day. In fact it is better to clean your teeth carefully and properly even once every day than to clean poorly or anyhow many times a day. Very often patients come into the clinic and complain –"Oh, I've got bad teeth". And by this they mean they have a lot of fillings in their mouth. I don't have a problem with fillings as long as the mouth and teeth are cleaned every day. In fact a mouth with lots of fillings indicates to me that the individual has been conscious of his/her mouth. I would rather a mouth full of fillings but clean than one with no fillings but dirty and full of bugs and thick plaque. I always liken a dirty mouth to eating out of a plate (the plate you use every day) without washing the plate in between meals. What surprises me is especially the number of teenagers and young adults who profess not to brush their teeth although they eat every day! How ic-ch-hy can you get??? And they dress up so seductively and think they are prima donnas. If only the guys knew—the prima donna with icchy mouth. All you need really is just brushing the teeth and mouth whenever you are ready to step out. And a little flossing will not hurt— but we'll get to flossing later. It surprises me to note that the quest for clean teeth is more of a habit and a culture in many African and developing countries compared to North America and other developed countries and yet the latter have all the paraphernalia to keep their teeth clean. Maybe it is because the African culture teaches the youth to use the chewing stick or sponge to clean or brush their teeth before "touching the mouth with food in the morning" and these chewing herbal accoutrements have anti-inflammatory ingredients.

Gum Disease, Tooth Sensitivity And Root Cavities

At some stage in the progression of periodontal disease, the gum recedes (recession) or moves to a position below (the lower teeth) and above the original gum line (in upper teeth). As has already been said, mere old age may also cause this condition of recession but not necessarily with a preceding periodontal infection. Improper tooth brushing may be the cause of this state of recession. This recession of the gum exposes a section of the root nearest to the crown of the tooth. NOTE: the tooth has a "crown" (or the white part that you see), the "root" on the bottom under the gums like the root of a tree, and the middle part (called the 'neck') joining these two separate parts.

In some individuals this exposure leads to tooth sensitivity in the exposed 'neck' region. Not only can recession cause root sensitivity; it also predisposes the exposed root section to collect plaque and start the root part of the tooth to decay ('root caries'). The sensitive areas of the root can be treated either with a filling or with applications of desensitizing medications. There are very well known toothpastes especially formulated to treat root sensitivity. Fluoride applications are also used to combat both root sensitivity and root decay. These various agents desensitize the root surfaces of teeth by mechanically and physically blocking the tiny exposed 'nerve' holes on the surface of the tooth structure, hence isolating and protecting the tooth nerve from the tooth environment.

Pregnancy-Induced Gingivitis And Cavities

It appears that during pregnancy the mother's gums are more susceptible to various oral assaults, this being directly related to elevated hormone levels at this period. Because of this increased probability of inflammatory gingival (gum) changes, pregnant mothers should be particularly mindful of their oral health. Personally, I feel that all young women of child-bearing age should have their mouths checked and cleaned every six months and kept clean henceforth. This way one cannot be caught unawares and where the pregnancy catches one by surprise, (surprise, huh!) an examination with teeth and gum cleaning should be done soon after with proper professional consultation and a good home care regimen instituted.

I hate to be sexist but it seems to me therefore that women of child-bearing age should constantly have their teeth and gums checked by their dentist. I must, however add here that most studies have shown that although women generally have cleaner mouths and better general oral health compared to men, for some reason they also tend to have more cavities than men.

Less dramatic but similar effects on the gums are also observed in oral contraceptive users. Because of this tendency of oral contraceptives to exacerbate or worsen gingivitis or gum infections, women on birth control pills should also have their mouths checked at reasonable intervals, like every six months and habitually keep their mouths clean.

What has not been proven or studied is the belief among some women that pregnancy destroys their teeth. Many a woman has reported to the dentist that her teeth started 'going' as a result of her pregnancies. Some mothers have jokingly stated that they've lost a tooth for each baby they've had. This may be a direct result of the pregnant condition or else a consequence of neglect once pregnant. Or else because some women acquire rather 'weird' cravings or "pica habits' when pregnant, it is possible that during these periods in their life they tend to indulge in and crave diets that predispose them to getting cavities. My mother, bless her soul, had a predilection for pieces of mud off the rain-washed walls of sod houses back home in Africa. Now that I think of it, it is probably a naturally indirect way of supplementing her calcium supply? But how she came to acquire a craving for this particular stuff beats my imagination. I wonder if the doctor who delivered me had to scrape mud off me before spanking me?

Although it is just possible that hormonal influences could account for the observed increases in decayed teeth in some women during pregnancy, the exact mechanism has not yet been defined. But whether this is circumstantial is yet to be proven. But is it possible that the hormones, because of the growing baby, can remove calcium from mother's teeth whilst building the teeth and bones of the baby, and would render these women more susceptible to tooth decay? Food for thought, huh?

AIDS And Periodontal Disease

We've been made to understand, although with a question mark, that one does not get the AIDS virus from kissing a known carrier.

But from the foregoing discussion, if A is kissing someone with the aids virus when A has a severe periodontal (gum) disease, it seems obvious to me that A may be dangerously exposing him/herself to getting the virus. Periodontal disease with bleeding gums and pocket formation from infected gums offer an easy entrance into the blood stream. During the kissing process, it is obvious that mixing of body fluids do occur and copious amounts of the virus can get a facilitated access into the unsuspecting, previously unexposed individual. This is my take of the situation and hopefully may be tested in due course. The same may apply to having oral sex with an AIDS carrier. Again, oral sex, if A is the one 'giving', it seems to me, can be an even more serious enabling process. The virus in the semen or from the vagina from B will find access to A's blood stream through the opened gingival sulcus alongside the infected gums just as easily as has been determined in heterosexual relationships that have ended up with the transmission of the virus. Again, this is just logical conjecture and may be shown to be true or false with more research. In all cases therefore a condom will offer a logical protection.

Prevention and Treatment of Gum Diseases

Good Home Care Practices—Brushing and Flossing

The initial stages of gum disease (gingivitis) can easily be prevented or if already started be treated by proper and diligent home care practices. Because it is almost painless in these early states you may not notice the gradual onset of redness or puffiness and the only sign may be the occasional occult (slight) bleeding when brushing or flossing.

The simple trick is not to let plaque remain in your mouth for more than a day unmolested. You miss BRUSHING and FLOSSING for one day and you are giving plaque and calculus their first ticket to the party and giving them the chance to gain a foothold in your mouth. It is that simple. While brushing will remove plaque and food debris form the more accessible or the exposed areas of the mouth, flossing (done with a piece of thread) removes plaque and food particles hiding in between the teeth where most brush bristles will not reach, no matter what the toothbrush says.

If you want to challenge the usefulness of flossing, try this test. Brush your teeth in your normal everyday manner. After this try flossing in between the teeth and see if you won't still remove some food debris and plaque left lodging somewhere. I have always been surprised how, no matter how ably I have brushed my own teeth, that I still can dislodge some remaining food debris and plaque, small, maybe, but still important finding since I was so confident I had removed everything. It is often stated that if you brush but don't floss you are doing only half the job. Maybe not half, but at least the work would not be completely finished yet.

And flossing is ESPECIALLY USEFUL in many initial stages of bad breadth.

Mouth irrigating devices with water jets are useful adjuncts to good home care of the mouth but do not replace good old brushing and flossing. They can be useful where you do not have your brush and floss with you but should never be used as substitutes. They may give you a fresh feeling in the mouth, I am sure.

Since you can never brush away 'calculus' or 'tartar', as the hardened or calcified plaque is called, it behoves anyone with any amount of tartar to seek the services of the dental professional. These appointments become imperative and should be made for every three to six months depending upon your susceptibility (how fast you form tartar).

Only the dental professional can diagnose early periodontal disease. With the aid of x'rays and a probing instrument inserted gently between each tooth and its surrounding gums in an orderly fashion the dental provider can detect any increase in the otherwise healthy shallow crevices between the tooth and the gum. X'rays also help detect any changes in the normal bone height and any beginning bone destruction. The sites in the mouth most susceptible to calculus formation, as has already been mentioned, are especially the inside (tongue side) of the lower front teeth and the cheek side of the top back teeth (molars).

In spite of the best home care and all the TLC (tender loving care) we give to our teeth, some of us still form tartar, especially in the more susceptible sites like the inside of the lower front teeth. This can easily be removed at the dentist's. There, the dental professional uses both hand scrapers, and ultrasonic instruments (scalers) which cut the cleaning time considerably by vibrating the tartar off the teeth.

Periodontal disease can be facilitated by other factors and should be treated whenever noted. Some of these factors are:

1. Crowns ('caps') that don't fit well on the teeth. This condition allows leakage of saliva alongside the edges of the crown and start tooth decay around and underneath the cap.
2. Dental fillings that are packed too full inside the tooth and spill over into the gums (overhang);
3. Uneven meeting or crooked positioning of the upper and the lower teeth (the 'bite') can facilitate periodontal disease.

All these problems can be taken care of at the 'gum treatment' appointment which is still erroneously grouped together with "tooth polishing" as "cleaning" by many dentists. Treating periodontal disease, although almost always starts with gum and teeth cleaning, is more than cleaning or polishing the teeth, since it involves some more invasive procedures as 'scaling' and/or 'root planing' which 'clean not just the teeth but essentially cleans also the diseased gums (diseases pockets) lining the gums AND the root surfaces. Usually another appointment is scheduled in three to four months' time to assess the effectiveness of the treatment. If some of the pockets are still present in some areas more (cleaning) scaling is done in order to rid the mouth of all remaining pockets and debris.

The Periodontist

Where a periodontal problem has not responded well to routine care, the dentist may refer you to see a periodontist for consultation and further treatment where necessary. The periodontist is the dental specialist in the care of the gums and supporting bone. He has, as all specialties go, years of extra schooling and experience that allow him to employ special techniques to treat more difficult or advanced periodontal problems.

Cleaning and polishing teeth

I go to all extent in my office, to differentiate between cleaning and 'cleaning'. In dentistry, "cleaning", as is generally practiced, comes in two forms:

1. There is the regular cleaning (prophylaxis) where the stained teeth are polished with a polishing paste. This is generally done in a reasonably 'clean' mouth with mild gum disease but where food debris and stains exist.

2. Then, there is the other kind of 'cleaning' (appropriately termed "scaling") which involves removing the foreign, unwanted hard deposits that have formed with time around the teeth and under the gums. The hard, encrusted, sometimes brown or black, rough deposits, that usually form around the neck of the teeth, are removed with this all-inclusive scaling.

It is important for dental offices to differentiate between these two methods of cleaning when talking to patients because of the many important implications.

The first implication is that the fees for these two procedures are very different. Whereas the regular cleaning my cost you only a few dollars, the other 'cleaning' (scaling) can run you about 3-4 times the regular cleaning fee. The ultimate fee charged will depend on the extent of the tartar or calculus around the teeth and/or submerged under the gums, and how many units of time it takes to remove these, a unit of time being about fifteen minutes. In those with gum disease the 'cleaning' may involve taking the cleaning instruments down between the roots of the teeth AND the gum and sometimes even to clean the diseased bone that supports the teeth (this process called ROOT PLANING). Sometimes the dental professional may have to go about four to five millimeters down into this space to clean the area of all accumulated debris and pus. Because there may be a little discomfort associated with this phase of 'cleaning' the operator (dental professional, either the dentist or the hygienist) may decide to freeze or numb the teeth and the gums for this procedure to ensure a painless, more comfortable procedure.

The second implication is the known fact that some patients walk away from one of these cleanings complaining of "such a high cost for just a cleaning". Every time I have heard patients complain I've always asked if the cleaning was of the first or second variety. Of course most often the patient would not know a 'scaling' from Adam. Such misunderstandings just go to show how miserably we dentists have failed to communicate what we know and do for our patients.

Supposing it takes me the usual forty-five minutes to an hour to 'clean' or scale a moderately heavy collection of tartar from patient A. If one unit of scaling costs $40, it means the bill for A is $120 (45/15 x40). Add to this now the fee of say $30 for polishing the teeth after the scaling and A is into the three figure billing of $150. And most of the time polishing maybe done sometimes before as well as after a 'scaling' or 'root planing'. This is because 'prophylaxes', (and this has nothing to do with the condom), or tooth polishing, smoothens the tooth and delays or retards the initial formation of Debris or plaque (bug) that may develop into tartar.

The third implication is that generally dentists are so poor at communicating treatment plans to patients that patients see subsequent recalls for the scaling and root planning as a way to gouge more money from them. In many cases the teeth are in such poor shape 'gum-wise' that the provider will not be able to complete 'cleaning' the whole mouth in just one day.

You see, the mouth is divided into what are called four 'quadrants'. This simply means 'four sections' and in the case of a particularly heavy tartar collection it may take two or more cleaning sessions to complete all quadrants. The problem is that the patient will have to be asked to return to the office two or more times just to complete the prepared treatment plan or to assess the healing in three to four months' time to make sure the gums are healing fine and to see if the 'cleaning' is doing its job of preventing tartar and the other attendant bacterial debris. Many patients have been known to complain that they were at the dentists only a few months ago and will not show up for any appointment until their next check-up time in a year's time. So therein lies the problem of either poor communication, poor patient education or else pure ignorance.

5D. Other Mouth Problems

Bad Breath Or Halitosis

You are a lady talking to a gentleman you just met and you find the individual attractive and a prospective friendship material, the kind of companion you've been looking for and will be eager to keep. You never know, this may end up in a meaningful relationship. As you talk to him, you noticed a slight grimace on his face and he keeps looking away a lot as if distracted. You wonder who else is in the picture stealing his attention. And yet, there is no one around to explain his reluctance to look you in the face. As you attempt to make a crucial point he imperceptibly moves away. Just a little, as if avoiding your space. You notice soon that he is holding his breath, his lips tightened together and before you know it, is gasping for air. He turns around, hides his face momentarily and in the same instance, unbeknownst to you, he lets out and takes in a deep breath like a diver coming up for precious air before going under once again.

You know something is wrong, but can't put your finger on it. You begin to talk fast to hide your embarrassment but the more you talk the bluer he looks. The poor guy is holding his breath every chance he gets. At this point, he can only see your mouth moving. He can't stand it anymore. What a stream of odoriferous stench! He makes some fast and inaudible excuse to see you again soon. With a quick about turn he takes in one deep, welcoming, and preciously exhilarating breath of escape. He is probably lost for good!

Not exactly what you had planned but, oh, there is the next time. There will be no next time. Not until you visit your friendly dentist!

Although bad breath has many causes, I would start looking for solutions, initially at least, from the dentist. With the exception of certain internal problems, with respiratory or alimentary canal disease being the two main reasons, dental causes are usually the first to seek help to eliminate. If the dental consultation does not work, and you are still exuding this constant concoction of putrefied exhale, then I would visit the physician next, and fast.

Causes of Bad Breath

First, everything should be in a gaseous form if you are going to smell it. Although bad breath is a result of putrefied, rotten products what you smell are sulphur products in a gas form. These are sulphides like hydrogen sulphide (from rotten eggs) and mercaptans — all are compounds containing sulphur. Hence what you smell are exhaled sulphur-containing gases called VSCs— Volatile Sulphur Compounds.

Most of bad breath originates or are formed initially in the mouth — about 85% of bad breath has its cause from the mouth. Let's go over the main causes of bad breath:

a. Haliphobia: Some people may think they have bad breath even though they don't. These people have a very low esteem of themselves and may blame their inadequacies or bad luck on the thought that it is because they have bad breath. These people will need reassurance from friends and the dental team to understand that they don't have any bad breath problem. It may just be a problem with self-esteem and lack of confidence.

b. Some foods: Some foods just smell bad and will give you bad breath when you consume them. Typical are my own favourite foods: garlic and onions. These are terrific foods but alas, they give breath problems, too. The other examples are other people's favourites — smoking (tobacco) and drinking (alcohols, wine also on occasion).

c. Medications: Some drugs will leave their "smell" on your breath the way some penicillins leave their scent in your urine. For a example, asthmatics taking ventolin puff may find this a problem but this is not bad breath. Your partner should understand that the smell on your breath is from the medication you are on.

However, some drugs cause bad breath because they actually cause dry mouth (xerostomia) as side effect. A dry mouth will smell because there is not saliva or spit to dilute the products the germs are constantly producing in your mouth. Of course, you know that there are millions of germs in your mouth, in everybody's mouth. Oh, don't worry about that, because that is not the problem. It is when you don't clean your mouth often or lubricate your mouth enough or properly that the germs predominate and fill your mouth with their "germ shit'. Yes, you can look at bad breath emanating from infected gums as germ 'shit." Now, how does that revelation make you feel, huh?

Some of the drugs that may cause dry mouth as their side effects, and therefore bad breath, are: hypertension drugs, sedatives and tranquilizers, anti-depressants and anti-histamines (decongestants).

d. Some diseases: diabetes has a smell that goes with that problem; cancer of the liver, kidney (like kidney failure); BUT CONSTIPATION DOES NOT CAUSE BAD BREATH!!! Some respiratory diseases, especially upper respiratory problems and gastrointestinal problems may cause bad breath; hence belching or even throwing up (vomiting) can impart some bad breath but constipation does not.

e. Sinus infections: infections in the nose or around the facial sinuses will give bad breath either from the nose or the mouth. Hence, dentists who deal with bad breath problems work very closely with Ear, Nose and Throat (ENT) specialists.

f. Tooth decay or rotten teeth: are you surprised? Sure, tooth decay harbours all these decayed (remember the words —"decay" "rotten") teeth. Yes, a tooth decay contains rotten and decayed tooth products filled with germs eating away unchecked. Be warned and fix all your decayed rotten teeth if you want to get rid of that bad breath problem.

g. The tongue: the top of the tongue is covered with a patch of papillae or little projections like a carpet or a field of grass. Hiding between these little projections are your friendly germs doing their own thing at your expense. The tongue is therefore a major, major cause of bad breath in the mouth and you are admonished to really clean your tongue as part of your daily oral hygiene procedures. There are tongue-scrapers just for this job and you may ask your friendly dentist. Or you can even just use the spoon to clean and scrape the top and back of the tongue.

h. Gum disease — Of all the causes of bad breath this is probably the biggest cause of them all.

Tooth decay, the tongue and gum disease together form 85% of the causes of bad breath from the mouth. Large, exposed cavities harbor a potpourri of bacteria and food debris and are a brew of an odoriferous (smelly) mixture. Bacteria can infiltrate a damaged, cracked or broken filling and thereby start a hidden and unattractive incidence of bad breath. Gum disease, as has been discussed above, is most often a sure and a favourite site. Only when all the cavities have been restored (fixed) and the gum disease treated with good home care regime in place and religiously maintained would I consider checking with the physician if the bad breath persists.

Testing for bad breath

The difficulty with bad breath is that virtually everybody notices it but no one around you is prepared to let you in on the secret. Like love, it is always in the air, and like love, many are unwilling to commit. Hence, to find out if people have been keeping their distance lately on account of something you 'said' and you want to play the sleuth, here are some simple tests you can administer yourself.

1. Cup hands tightly together, trying not to allow any space between the two opposing pinky (little) fingers as if you are going to pray. And in any case if you don't pray, this maybe just the time to start! Now cover your mouth and nose placed against the thumbs between the tightly cupped hands, trying not to allow any space anywhere that will allow air out of this

secret tipi (triangular-shaped structure) you've just erected with your hands. Now breath through your mouth into this space with a steady but deep Haaaaa — just like the doctor ordered. Now sniff after each breath of the Haaa. If your breath smells bad to you, it probably does to your unsuspecting neighbours as well.

2. If you have a face mask it works even better still. Instead of cupped hands, put the face mask on and adjust the strap nice and tight around your head. Breath through your mouth into the face mask and smell your breath as you breathe out. If you have bad breath this will show you immediately.

3. Get yourself a dental floss, even though up till now the only floss you've heard of is "The Mill On The Floss" (a favourite literature book in "Secondary" School). Any drug store will have the dental floss. Stores in some African communities may not have the floss. By this time you probably do not know what the heck this silly strand of cotton is for so go at it easy and gently. We don't want to spook you now since you will soon have to adopt it and make it a bosom friend.

And we don't want you to hang yourself with it although by this time you would feel like hanging yourself for letting things go this far. Using the two hands and in any which way you can, gently pass the floss between any two teeth. Pull the thread (from now on 'floss' to you!) between your teeth. If the mouth smells bad after this exercise or if the area of floss in contact with the teeth smells bad, just as easily you have bad breath. You might even be able, even for a first timer, to dislodge some gunk out from between the teeth.

If you want a very romantic evening on this night out please stay away from foods listed below — at least just for today. After that you can wallow in them to your heart's content. As far as I can see, the only use these food items are to you breath-wise is to indulge in them just before your visit to your dentist to punish him for charging you a leg and an arm for that root canal.

Foods To Avoid On A date

1. **Garlic:** as has been mentioned, garlic is good for your health but this is one time it may prove your undoing. If you are Ukrainian, this one time switch to another nationality for heaven's sake and go garlic free—it is environmentally UN-friendly. Depending on the amount eaten and the time of ingestion, garlic can stay on your breath for a whole day. The ONION is the other offending food item in this category. Oh No, you say. And how I love them on my hamburgers! But then if you go for hamburgers on a romantic evening (and you are not a student or a teenager) then maybe, just maybe, you may have a reason to blow on this cheapskate all the bad breath you've got.

2. Other Ukrainian favourites like prepared delicatessen meats, some or all of which may also contain garlic, are a no-no before that date or interview: pastrami, salami, pepperoni and garlic sausages;

3. I love **cheese**, especially the fort or the strong, old variety, and that may explain why I never had dates when I was a student at the university. Just like garlic, cheese is a healthy food but 'some are more equal than others' and are not meant for you at certain critical moments in your life — like moments that call for a close tête a tête with your girlfriend or spouse. Stay away therefore from strong types like: the blue cheese, Camembert and the Roquefort. Greek salad, great as it may be, unfortunately has two of the above undesirable ingredients of cheese and garlic. Be warned — don't go Greek and don't go Ukrainian if your life depends on it. Not tonight, anyway.

4. Do you notice that so far all the items that have been discussed are some of the good things in life: and who said life was easy? Not on your life. You may not like fish but I do, and as you just guessed, some fish preparations belong to the to-be-avoided-at-all-cost category. The smell some (usually canned) fish leave on your breath may not be that strongly repulsive but enough to make some people, like my kids, wanna puke (throw up,

vomit). But then, my kids puke at anything anyway. Do not have anchovies, sardines and tuna for lunch if you want to catch the big one today.

5.   Don't you wanna scream at all the good things we are not supposed to eat these days? As if the list is not enough already, here are some more: coffee and many alcoholic beverages, whisky, beers and some wines. Maybe your best bet tonight is vodka; I hear they don't smell. I wonder if that is true! Hmmm. And these beverages tend to leave you with a stench mouth in the morning-after as well.

6.   And talking about stench mouth, what does it better than cigarettes? 'Nobody does it better', to steal a saying from the great romantic himself, a James Bond movie song. And not only will cigarettes kill you literally, but smoking really puts a damper on your romantic life. And not only does your mouth stink but your whole body can reek of the smoke a mile away. Its not exactly the sweet grass it is made out to be. An interesting observation is that some people actually keep on smoking to cover up already existing problem of mouth odour. This way you can blame it on the cigarette not on poor oral hygiene practices. If you really want to be conniving or empathizing, then you should have your partner also take on the habit of smoking. That way you both smell bad and he/she will not be repulsive and none of you will be the wiser.

How Not To 'Take His/Her Breath Away'

There are a few things one can do in spite of breaking one of these cardinal rules of breath-saving.

1.   The first and foremost, use your toothbrush. You can eliminate many fowl smells from the mouth simply by brushing the teeth and gums after such a momentary lapse into the no-no food habits. If it does not do you any good it will at least get rid of the unsightly piece of lettuce in between your front teeth after

that Greek salad. Even though some of these foods have their own inherent bad odour, brushing the teeth and the gums after the meal will eliminate the myriads of bugs now clamouring to share the food remains left in the plaque-covering on your teeth.

2. And whilst you are at it brush your tongue as well as the teeth and gums. We tend to forget to brush the tongue as a matter of fact. For some people, asking them to brush the tongue is like asking the anorexic to eat peas. But the tongue is a big factor if one wants to eliminate mouth odours. The tongue, as has already been mentioned, can harbor plaque and remnants of food. This combination is the witch's brew and a prescription for a stench mouth. These bugs hide in their little huts and after every meal go around jubilating — 'stench mouth, anyone'?

    If you are like me, brushing the tongue will always excite the gagging reflex. But like all things in this world that is worth fighting for, onward we must go, gag or no gag. And isn't it nice to know you are not the only one? Then do as I do. Brush all parts of the tongue real fast for a few seconds, then cool it, and wait for the next good time, which for me is a good minute before I can compose myself for another torture. Then I get in there hard and vigorous for another few seconds and cool it once more. After a third attempt at this game of hide and seek, I am clean, but not to mention the tears and the now red-shot eyes from the attendant retching.

3. Use a good, scented toothpaste. The toothpaste will definitely help clean away the smelly plaque. Other toothpastes, like the baking-soda types now on the market, will actually aid in eliminating some of the odour in the mouth. And if you don't habitually put a dish of baking soda in your refrigerator to remove the smell, now you know. In the developed world like North America this may sound primitive; the problem is, you may not even find the stuff, but if you were to get your hands on it, wood charcoal powder does the same trick as baking soda. In many African countries where wood charcoal is a popular fuel for cooking, powdered charcoal is used to brush the teeth, both

for its whitening properties and for the fact that it eliminates bad odour in the mouth. The problem is if not well rinsed out you will have some of the black powder sticking in between your teeth for your troubles. I routinely used this in my youth back home in Ghana.

4. Rinse out your mouth often. Whenever you can't brush, at least rinse if only for a brief reprieve (good for about 30 minutes). After lunch at work you can go into the washroom and rinse out the mouth with copious amounts of water, swishing vigorously each time. Three vigorous attempts with copious amounts of water will do the trick to dislodge any remaining food particles sticking on the teeth.

5. If you really cannot rinse the mouth because all these years you have not learnt how to do it, or you may be at a restaurant where you just cannot get up for the washroom (I just cannot think of any reason why not but for argument's sake, or unless only an outhouse is available where you happen to be, like in my village, or you are lunching with your boss and you feel shy to leave), then take a mouthful of water from your drinking glass, swish the mouth by moving the water all around the teeth, and do the one thing you never wanted to do in your life— swallow it, bugs and all. Unless you can spit it out in the sand under the table by your boss' shoes. To tell you the truth I never could swish and swallow until very recently when I found myself at this party where I could not get up to go wash my mouth after the meal.

6. Learn to gargle as part of your daily oral hygiene practice. If you have bad breath, a gargle with a medicated mouthwash containing chlorhexidine or other effective anti-bacterial or anti-plaque agent will do. Some mouthwash preparations— like Listerine, although it does not taste good, and that is why even bugs can't stand it—, have active ingredients that will actually kill the odour-producing bugs in the mouth. Then the flavouring also helps reduce the bad smell emanating from your direction, like from your mouth. You can also buy the scented mouth spray which comes in a small vial sold by Avon, if you

are anticipating a very short but odour-free date, for about thirty minutes.

7.   Chew gum, especially a sugarless gum. Aside of getting rid of some mouth odour on account of the flavouring, chewing gum will also eliminate some smelly food debris from the teeth. As an added bonus, one particular sugar-less gum (with xylitol as the sugar substitute) actually promotes the reversal of some beginning, small cavities. Since bad breath can be caused by dry mouth as when fasting or going without food for long periods of time, chewing something like gum will cause constant flow of saliva and help eliminate the bad odour, unless you are barred while fasting even to chew gum.

8.   I could not believe it when I heard that chewing certain herbs and spices can give you sweet-smelling breath, but it makes sense. If it smells good somewhere else it probably will work in the mouth. Parsley is supposed to help freshen the breath so next time at the supermarket get a bunch for your brunch— hey, I can be a poet—a bunch for your brunch!!! Ha! Cloves, fennel and anise are also in this category. Chew on these when it is time to camouflage the suspected mouth odour. By the same reasoning, chewing a mint will camouflage the sneaky odours from your mouth area for as long as the mint lasts. This, however, can be an expensive habit since you will have to eat a lot of it, and one that, if it becomes a habit, will land you at your dentist's door willy-nilly. You may be promoting tooth decay, on the account of the sugar in the mint, and land you from the frying pan into the fire.

9.   Use your hands: In my youthful days in Ghana, I used to see my uncles do this every time after meals when we were working at the farm at my grandfather's cottage. They would rinse the mouth first and then retaining a little bit of water in the mouth, scrub the teeth both on the outside and the inside, using the first finger. It may not do a good job but it will help clean some of the remnants of food debris off the teeth.

10. I don't know if this agent is still on the market but it used to be available in the United States a few years back. This superb agent was called 'OXFRESH' and boy, was it ever great! Go to your nearest dealer or ask your dentist and he may be able to get you samples if they are still on the market. Oxyfresh came in many preparations but what you are after are the Oxyfresh toothpaste and the mouthwash. These agents, actually attack the sulphur compounds produced by the bugs in the mouth and leave you with odour-free mouth for that lucky date;

11. And as has already been mentioned, no matter what you do the bad breath will not go away if you have decayed teeth in your mouth. You should have all tooth decay or cavities filled if you are thinking of eliminating bad breath.

12. Avoid eating a lot of proteins like meats and dairy products (milk); frequent intake of carbohydrates is more helpful. Also, if you have problem with bad breath avoid fasting since fasting can cause bad breath if prolonged. Or don't go on a date if you are fasting. Frequent intakes of carbohydrates, even of small amounts with chewing, will help rid you of the accursed mouth odour.

13. If you can get your hands on it, chewing this exotic —tiger nuts— is normally an antidote for mouth odour. The other good stuff is sugar-cane. But you have to have good teeth to chew this sweet stick. Cucumber juice is also said to be refreshing and heals diseased gums, leaving your mouth smelling good.

Consult Your Physician If Bad Breath Persists

If you find that all these offer temporary relief and are only band-aid solutions, which I suspect they will be since the underlying cause may not have been attacked, then make haste to your dentist pronto. Persistent mouth odour after the dentist and all the above precautions mean you may have trouble somewhere else other than the mouth. You may be passing odourous gases but not from the usual oral channel.

Some other medical problem may be the cause of your mouth odour: cancer, dehydration, gastrointestinal and/or respiratory problem. Then your dentist should refer you to the physician. As earlier observed, some medications can impart specific odours to your breath. At least, if you knew it was from the medication, you can rest free, knowing there is nothing seriously wrong. Personally, I have come across people with mouth odour emanating from constant puffs of mouth applications of their aerosol asthmatic medications. At least you will have a reasonable excuse.

Wisdom Teeth Problems

Wisdom teeth, thus named for reasons only known to history, start forming in the jaw bone in females as early as the 13th age but do not generally appear in the mouth till around the age of 17-19 years. In typical African countries, girls have been observed to have their first wisdom teeth at the age of 13 years. I presume for mankind, therefore, one reaches the age of accountability with the eruption of these teeth since they are the last teeth to make their appearance in the mouth. One rule of thumb: if your wisdom tooth stays down in the jaw till after the age of around 23 to 25 years, it probably will never come through. One should probably not say 'never' but there is a lot of evidence for that. Adults in their fourties who have had the tooth in front of the impacted wisdom tooth removed a long time ago and there is therefore plenty of room for it to erupt have realized in the end, that the wisdom tooth has still not properly erupted into place like it should.

In some people, these teeth do not form at all, in which case the individual only has a total of 28 teeth. It is said that humans have 32 teeth but this is only in the lucky majority in whom these wisdom teeth form and erupt in the mouth. There are people in whom wisdom teeth will form but will decide not to show up completely and remain partly hidden in the bone, every once in a while making their presence felt but never showing their full face or heads in the mouth area. When this happens, we say the tooth is impacted.

Wisdom teeth, to most people in the industrialized world, are pure nuisance. In the more ancient populations, usually in the industrially developing world, there is most often enough room in the jaw for their complete eruption. Probably because of their relatively rough, raw diet and the amount of hard chewing involved, people in these third world societies have well developed jaw bones and exhibit a reduced tendency for the wisdom teeth to remain down in the jaw bone (that is, these populations have fewer 'impacted' wisdom teeth). In the relatively 'newer' societies, like in most western countries, the diet is so devoid of intense chewing that 'seeing' they are not needed, the wisdom teeth have decided to let sleeping dogs lie and just do no bother to erupt, a case of use and disuse atrophy? In actual fact, though, chewing has been shown to stimulate and encourage the growth of the jaw bone.

This does not mean you will develop healthy wisdom teeth if you moved to Africa. The eruption of wisdom teeth probably has a hereditary component and is presumably in the genes so that no amount of coaxing will bring it out, no matter where you decide to live.

Wisdom teeth can be a nuisance, pure and simple. For some reason, and this is probably not connected with anything, but I often noticed an increased incidence of wisdom teeth problems especially during the Christmas season. There were a few individuals who came for palliative treatment (just to ease the pain) every Christmas season on account of their wisdom teeth. Interestingly, they never bothered to have these teeth removed and sure enough, they were in the office the next Christmas with infected wisdom teeth. One lady did this for three consecutive Christmases and probably still has the wisdom teeth.

Impacted wisdom teeth (those that decide to stay down in the bone and not show up in the mouth) can present a variety of problems. In most cases, the overlying gum surrounding the partially erupted tooth becomes infected and presents with chewing difficulties. A palliative treatment may be to have the overlying gum removed so that chewing is not painful or else the tooth may be removed when the infection subsides. Your dentist will give you the options and will let you know if and just when you need to continue with the requisite treatment. Once the partially erupted wisdom tooth starts bothering you, however, it will keep doing this every once in a while until something is done, or definitive treatment is given.

I know of one particular incident where this 30-years old man had visited the eye specialist, a neurosurgeon, an ear-nose-and-throat specialist all with headaches that did not respond to any treatment given. Somewhere at the end of his rope his physician, as a last resort, suggested to the patient to see a dentist. When I saw him this gentleman had an impacted wisdom tooth high high up in the tuberosity (the jaw bone behind the last top teeth) on the right side. His problems were over once this tooth was identified and removed.

If you have pains in the jaw, which comes not necessarily with chewing; the whole face or jaw aches anytime in the day or at night; a kind of dull but persistent pain; a pain the site of which you cannot exactly pin-point; a persistent headache; if you have some or all of these see your dentist since it could very well be a wisdom tooth.

There is an on-going debate whether impacted wisdom teeth should be removed once noticed. I adopt a more pragmatic approach: if the impacted tooth: 1. does not bother you; 2. if from examination there is no associated pathology (ie. no infection or abnormal growth in its surroundings that looks suspicious), or 3. If your orthodontist does not feel they should be removed to alleviate possible future crowding, I leave it alone. However, it should be checked at every regular visit at the dentist and whenever there is the slightest indication of a problem that would be the time to do something. To remove it routinely and purely as a preventive measure does not warrant the time and money involved, and to my thinking, the possible post-operative suffering that sometimes is associated with this surgery. But then to each his own, and if you decide to go that route by all means do so.

CHAPTER 6

DENTISTRY AND PAIN CONTROL

Pain, euphimistically speaking, is either a dentist's friend or his enemy. It is his friend because that is the one major factor that brings many people to his office. In a rural dental practice about 70 per cent of the patients fall in this category and only go to the dentist when there is pain; until the next episode of a toothache. The problem with dentistry is, a person comes in to have the pain relieved only to be met with another form of pain, momentary and negligible though it may be. It is probably the only profession that, in an attempt to remove pain, produces one in the process. I guess you can say we fight fire with fire, huh.

Next to financial reasons, fear of dental work ranks very high in the reasons people give for avoiding dental visits. Simultaneously, whilst pain is a friend when it brings people into the office, it is also the enemy in the sense that many stay away from the dentist. It is estimated that the biggest single factor may be fear and that three out of every four people experience some dental anxiety. In spite of the fact that modern dentistry can be virtually painless and has made great strides in developing pain-control methods, dentistry still has a tough time shaking this simple reputation.

But really, the dentistry practiced today is a vast improvement over that in the days of 'Painless Parker', as many seniors over sixty-five will well attest to. And yet with this much improvement, the public still seeks dental treatment with disdain.

Dentistry has therefore a love-hate relationship with the public, love when they can't stay away from its clutches, and hate when everything is right with them dentally. Or is it the other way around? Hence, there is an ambivalence towards the dental profession which no other profession on earth enjoys, with the exception of the fear reserved for the traditional medicine men who go around in many African villages circumcising young males without anesthetic. If you think dental treatments hurt, try having a circumcision done with a razor blade which has been used on five other 'patients' before you without any prior anesthetic! Dentistry with freezing is a breeze compared to the circumcision experience.

Dental Needles and Local Anaesthetics

A dental treatment should not be as bad as it has been made to appear. Nowadays, needles are not used over and over as they used to be 'those days'. Each patient these days has a new, and a sharp needle which is disposed of after one use. In dentistry, the needles used are of the smallest and finest caliber. The most prevalent needles are 'Gauges' 25, 27 and 30 (the smaller and finer the needle or the bore, the bigger the gauge. Hence the biggest Gauge size, # 30, has the smallest bore). Most dental offices use the popular gauge 27, and a few dentists like myself use gauge 30 because they profess it to be less painful. Using gauge 30, however, demands more attention to detail and a finer technique because it is very thin and can break if used injudiciously as compared to the other gauges. Although the 30 gauge is also blamed for ineffective aspiration (a technique employed while giving the injection to make sure one is not injecting into a blood vessel), many dentists have not found this to be a problem.

A patient has every right to indicate to the dentist if the freezing is not adequate enough for his/her comfort level. And a dentist should stop working and add some more anesthetic enough to provide a more comfortable session. The anesthetics used in dentistry are locally administered, in the sense that they are deposited in one region to numb just that area. Especially in the upper teeth, each tooth can in fact be anesthetized (frozen) just by itself. Because the lower jaw is a lot denser, it is more efficient in many cases to freeze groups of teeth since they happen to be supplied by the same bundle of nerves (i.e. the same one nerve goes to this group of teeth). Freezing one lower tooth by itself can be done a lot easier in children but less so in some adults and even then with some teeth but not with others. This specific site technique is more useful with children because the bone is young and less dense.

I remember a gentleman who wanted to have a tooth in the middle of the lower jaw—just behind the right lower eye tooth—removed. As I was preparing the site for the injection, (which for lower teeth is way back of the mouth behind the wisdom tooth) he was observant enough to ask me if I can anaesthetize one tooth at a time then how come I was preparing an area quite out of the way of the offending tooth. I had to stop and with a note book illustrated to him how the anatomy of the lower jaw works.

In the mouth each tooth has its own nerve. Along with the nerve are also the vessels that carry blood to the tooth to keep it alive and well. This group or bundle of nerve and blood vessels travel through the jaw bone and as it goes on its merry way gives off branches to each tooth. Just like the drinking pens in a pig farm. Some teeth have stray nerves coming to them from nearby nerves as well so they have multiple enervation (supplied by different nerves). All teeth therefore have certain specific sites from where they can be reached and "frozen". And because of the multiple enervation of certain teeth the dentist has to anesthetize or "freeze" these teeth in two or more places to achieve adequate anesthesia.

The Freezing Medication and Your Medical History

These days many dentists routinely apply a topical anesthetic initially to the site where a tooth will be later anesthetized (frozen). This is in order to numb the area (like jiffy) before the actual freezing is done. This practice has gone a long way to making dental freezing a lot easier and less painful. Usually the topical anesthetic applied is a stronger concentration of the same anesthetic (freezing) to be employed later and comes either as a spray, solution, gel or ointment.

The freezing medication itself comes as a solution in a small, thin glass or plastic vial (called carpoule) which fits perfectly into the metal (or sometimes plastic) syringe. The syringe with the carpoule sitting inside it is then fitted with the needle for the injection. So the 'needle', as dental patients know it, consists really of three parts: the syringe or carrier, the carpoule of anesthetic that fits inside a slot in the syringe, and the (say, 27 gauge) needle which fits at the end of the syringe carrier.

There are many different types of freezing medications, but they are only different in their duration, the amounts needed (the different dosages), the family of chemicals and the specific additives which perform different functions. Hence, a dentist may use one type for the diabetic and another for an individual with no indicated medical condition. One type of anesthetic used will stay around the site in the mouth where the dentist would be working for about an hour whereas another type will persist for two to three hours, depending upon the expected duration of the procedure, the age and the medical condition of the patient

Hence the importance of a patient giving all known medical history to the dental professional who will be conducting the health interview, whether it is the receptionist, the dental assistant or the dentist himself. You may think your being allergic to pineapples is not a pertinent medical history to be revealed in the dental office until you later learn that some of the topical anesthetics the dentist uses have a pineapple flavouring. Or you have been bleeding incessantly for two hours after that tooth was extracted (removed) because you did not think it useful or necessary to tell the dentist that you had been taking aspirin for that toothache for the last two days. Aspirin, as one of its many functions, also prevents blood from clotting. In fact, some dental schools teach their students not to remove a tooth when the patient had taken aspirin in the course of the same day that they report for the extraction. The point of this discussion is that everything in your medical history could be important to the dentist and you should not sift through it and give only what you feel will be pertinent.

'Painless Parker'—The Painless Dentist

To give a relatively painless freezing a dentist employs a few known techniques. First, he should not rush it. It is important to take the necessary time to do it right. A rushed freezing usually ends with the patient "climbing the ceiling" (may hurt a lot) or the patient may grab the edge of the chair and make the knuckles so white they might break the chair. Taking about a minute for each carpoule is not wasting time. Some dentists feel that the faster they give the freezing, the more efficient and 'better dentists' they appear to the patients. I have never had a patient complaining because I took too long to do the freezing. The only problem has been that because I take 'longer' time to complete the anesthesia a few patients get the idea that I am putting in a lot of freezing. This, although is appreciated by many, may not go down well with those patients who want to appear "macho" sometimes to impress the female dental assistants. However, explaining that this slow and gentle technique is for their own good, that it is the only way I know how, and that I was still only using one carpoule and within the allowable dosage, settles even the persistent macho.

There are many advantages to a slow delivery of the local anesthetic solution.

1. Imagine putting water in a balloon. If done slowly and gently the balloon fills up nicely and the contents are distributed evenly all around inside the balloon. However, if the water is forcefully introduced into the balloon it would tend to burst prematurely. In the dental office the only thing that will be doing the bursting may be the chops of the dentist (from an irate patient— pow-w) if he/she does not do it slowly and gently!

2. When done, gently and slowly, the often attendant reaction resulting from the inadvertent introduction of the anesthetic solution into a blood vessel is usually mild or does not occur.

3. The patient can, as it were, be titrated while injecting and introducing the medicine slowly so that any untoward immediate reaction can be noticed and forestalled forthwith.

4. You do not really waste any time. In fact this minute has been well spent because if you have to give a second carpoule, by the time you get around to it the first freezing would already have started working and the second one is then peanuts, kapish?

And by the way some patients may shy away from asking for more freezing mainly because they think subsequent freezing may 'hurt' just as much as the first one. Given time, any more freezing, if you need more than one, is just a piece of cake. For argument sake, you can have as many as five 'freezings' and all subsequent ones after the first one will not be felt.

Of course a new, sharp needle is a must. Then it is also a good idea to exploit the useful initial numbing effect of a topical anesthetic.

Music and Dentistry

If music be the fruit of love, play on. This was not said in jest. A well selected music for a dental office is indeed a panacea for the background cacophony of drills, suctions and piercing cries of unmanageable children that pervade the atmosphere of a typical dental office. And it soothes everyone's soul. I always say when asked by patients that the music I play is probably more for myself than for the patients. It helps 'cool me down' just as I hope it does the patient. Humming, singing, tapping or whistling to the music gets my mind off any other thoughts and wonderfully projects my attention solely to the work at hand. Try it – it may do wonders for you too. And it does not have to be only in the office. And you don't even have to be a dentist to use music while you work. I think husbands should encourage their housewives to work to music – get them a radio or these days buy an I-Pod.

This way house wives will be so cool, stress-free and happy that there will be no more complaining about nocturnal or headaches at night on the matrimonial bed. And there will be less depression in the world. I guarantee it.

Pain Control and The Dental Patient's Responsibility

The aim here is to build a relationship of trust between you and your dentist. The means to achieve this rapport is COMMUNICATION. This word has been bandied about since the 80s and yet we still seem to miss the message. If this book does not do anything for you, I hope it will at least encourage you to begin frank discussions about your anxieties towards dental treatments. DO NOT HIDE YOUR ANXIETIES. Speak out about your fears to the dentist or a staff member who hopefully will relay this important information to the dentist. As a dentist, I would rather a patient tells me openly how he/she feels about an impending dental work. And the dentist should treat this revelation with all seriousness. It is unfortunate but I have heard and actually seen some dental offices which have this sign at the reception area – "WE CATER TO COWARDS". This I feel is insensitive and disrespectful. Patients who are anxious about their dental work are NOT cowards. And how can such patients be open with you the dentist when you've already labeled them as cowards? Nobody, not even I, would admit to being a coward. As a dentist you are supposed to take the time to listen to your patient's concerns, learn about them, and gain their confidence so you can finally administer the appropriate treatment. How can you do that in all seriousness when these people are seen in such a derogatory manner? Dental patients should get the same empowerment that they have gained with their physicians. That does not mean they should be demanding or obstreperous but they should be able to understand what is being done to their bodies.

There is, however, cause for celebration. When asked the question: "When I think of going to the dentist, I think of pain", 58% of Canadians (1993) disagreed with the statement. Through sensitivity, compassion and ever improving pain control techniques dental teams can rise to the challenge of further eliminating the perception that dentistry and pain go hand in hand. The onus is now on dentists to work hard in this area of pain control so that future surveys would produce a 100% favourable response to that same question. That will then be truly a cause for celebration for dentists and patients alike.

CHAPTER 7

ROOT CANAL—AN UNDESERVED BUM RAP

Of all dental treatments the **root canal** (or 'endodontic tx'—endo = inside or within, 'dontic' = of the tooth) procedure has received the greatest bum rap and has provoked the most varied of horror stories by patients. A root canal procedure is basically the process where the dentist cleans inside the whole length of the tooth of all infected debris and then fills that cleaned space with a filling. The dentist does this cleaning treatment because the nerve inside the tooth is dead from one reason or another. Dentists in especially rural practices will probably attest to the unfortunate observation that a root canal treatment is one shunned by most prospective patients. Most of the time you end up removing the tooth which should have had root canal done because the owner does not wish to get a root canal treatment. I feel personally that many patients have conspired to give the root canal this bum rap to excuse them from a hidden underlying state of personal impecuniosity (lack of funds!). Which state is quite understandable and even to be sympathized with, but people for some reason do not want to come out straight and tell the dentist they cannot afford a treatment. Instead, all kinds of morbid stories have been concocted to explain why they may not want a root canal, even though they had never had one done.

A typical scenario—the dentist finishes with the examination of a tooth that has been bothering a patient 'on and off for about two months'. At the mention of a root canal treatment, the dentist is faced with a patient ready to fall off the chair shaking with all her might.

"No, not root canal", retorts our friendly patient.

The dentist asks, "Have you had any done before?"

"No, but I will rather have it (the tooth) removed", meaning, take the damn thing out! "But if you have never had one done then what is the problem?" The dentist observes, smiling with incredulity.

"I understand it hurts too much", is the curt reply. Straight and to the point.

"But if you've never had it, how do you know it's going to hurt"?, the dentist inquires, obviously baffled.

"My sister-in-law had it and she could not eat for a week. She said it hurt something fierce"! Others also would quote their relative, a neighbour or a friend who had one done and "they all reported it hurt". In my practice a few people said they had it done once and "it did not work so eventually the tooth had to be removed". Now how do you counter that argument?

Initial Warning!

When you have a tooth decay which is neglected and goes unattended (anywhere from a year to three years) it would tend to get bigger and deeper as the sugar bugs eat their way gradually further into the tooth structure in all directions. As this process continues the bugs finally reach the central part of the tooth where the canal with the bundle of nerves and blood connections to the tooth (pulp tissue or the 'nerve') is situated. The advancing zone of the tooth decay with its load of sugar bugs irritates the 'nerve' as the bugs continue producing toxins or irritants as part of their normal daily life processes. The nerve soon gets irritable and you start noticing this because that tooth now starts to ache. Actually, even before the 'nerve' region is reached there is an initial warning of sorts. The tooth may become sensitive to both hot and cold. At this stage the process may be reversible where the dentist will clean all the decayed material, apply a dressing over the top of the 'nerve' that is below the advancing decaying area and insert a filling over that to seal off the 'cavity' from any further insult. This treatment is usually enough to forestall any further problems if the tooth is not too far gone.

So, Then, What?

The dressing applied directly over the top layer of the 'nerve' acts as a mild 'healing' irritant to the area and in about six to eight weeks will generate a new layer of a different and a more resistant tooth structure which acts as insulation to the nerve underneath. This is why a new Filling may still show signs of the earlier reactions to both cold and hot foods for a while. The reaction should, however, subside with time until around six to eight weeks when to all intents and purposes the nerve should have appreciably healed.

The dentist goes by sight and therefore can only clean the decayed region until in his estimation all the softened or discoloured tooth has been removed. Sometimes, in his attempt to remove all the decay he may get to a point where the 'nerve' will be staring straight back at him. This 'caries exposure', where the decay is so deep that it has now unavoidably reached the outskirts of the 'nerve' region, is treated as described above with a dressing ('pulp cap') and allowed to heal.

If the infection has outreached the treatment and has spread more into the 'nerve' than was anticipated, the nerve is now infected and a root canal (or 'pulectomy') is indicated. This is also the case where a neglected, large, deep cavity finally develops with time and eats its way to the 'nerve' inside the tooth. At this point the infection is irreversible and only root canal can fix it. Or, of course the proverbial, 'pull it out'.

So What Is This Root Canal, Anyway?

Basically, a root canal treatment involves just cleaning all the infected and all dead and toxic products inside the tooth. Each tooth, like a straw in a bottle, has a space all the way down from the top to the bottom of the tooth. With a root canal treatment the cleaning goes beyond the regular filling which is usually limited only to the crown or the visible part of the tooth. In the root canal procedure the crown area as well as the infected 'nerve' area in the submerged root section of the tooth are cleaned and a filling placed to fill the clean space so created. Fine, handheld or ultrasonic cleaners (or 'files') are used to clean, 'ream' or 'file' inside the 'nerve' canal. To do this, x-rays are needed with which the dentist determines the exact length of the 'nerve' canal inside the tooth so that the filling will not be shorter or longer than the exact extent of the tooth canal.

Because the root canal procedure is time consuming, it is not uncommon for a typical appointment to run into an hour or more. And to ensure that all the infected debris is cleaned out the process may take two or more appointments in some cases. The rationale for the treatment is to clean out the infected products by gradually cleaning the canal and thereby removing any vestiges of infected material from within and around the walls of the space or canal.

But a root canal DOES NOT have to hurt. If the tooth is well anesthetized (frozen), it should be a breeze. Obviously the only time any dental procedure hurts is if the freezing is not adequate and that can be fixed with a deeper and proper freezing. The only instance I know can legitimately be said to be uncomfortable is where you have a 'hot tooth' on your hands. A 'hot tooth' is one with acute abscess, where the infected tooth is just beginning to cause swelling of the gums around or beside it and the patient comes to the office with a cold pack on the site of the tooth and in obvious pain. These teeth are often notoriously incapable of taking any freezing and it hurts so bad the patient cannot eat or bite on the tooth, even the tongue causes pain if it touches the tooth, and especially any warm stuff drives the owner crazy with pain. To relieve the pain the dentist may attempt to freeze it and open into the tooth to drain the accumulating toxic bacterial contents in the hopes of alleviating the pain. That CAN often be painful since the freezing will sometimes prove inadequate. At this early stage of the infection, there will not be any appreciable drainage anyway to provide relief since the infection is not that well organized (the body is still fighting the bugs and has not yet walled off the infection).

Most often the appropriate action would be for the dentist/physician to prescribe a potent painkiller together with antibiotics and leave for about 5 to 7 days to initiate some resolution of the condition.

Pulpotomy–Children's Root Canal, Sort Of

In baby teeth, as is also the case in new, recently erupted adult teeth, a tooth so infected may be conservatively and effectively treated. Here, the top layer of the presumably recently infected 'nerve' is removed (the process called 'pulpotomy) and appropriate medication applied and a filling placed on top of the dressing. In most situations where the initial aching symptoms bring the patient to the dentist soon enough this treatment is all that will be needed.

In the baby tooth, the tooth so treated with the top layer of the nerve removed and treated will stay in the mouth with no further problems until it is shed at the appropriate time. If this treatment does not work the infection progresses into an abscess and the tooth will then have to be removed and a spacer may have to be put in its place.

The newly erupted adult tooth which has undergone this treatment of pulpotomy will need a root canal in the future. This waiting period may be drastically reduced if this initial treatment of pulpotomy does not take; then a root canal is indicated a lot sooner.

"So when is a root canal indicated?" All the scenarios mentioned above will call for root canal treatment. Also, if a tooth gets fractured or broken in an accident and the 'nerve' is obviously exposed to the fluids and the bacteria (bugs) in the mouth, a root canal may be the treatment of choice. But the tooth should be fractured with obvious bleeding at the fractured surface. If the tooth is fractured but only a small piece came off without much bleeding it may not need a root canal and can be easily repaired with a filling. If there is blood on the surface (usually coming from the middle of the tooth) of the fractured tooth and not from the bruised gums, then you have a possible root canal treatment on your hands—or in your mouth. All abscessed teeth where the 'nerve' is frankly infected, with or without pus, will need root canal treatment.

Single-Visit Root Canal Therapy

The single-visit root canal procedure, where the whole treatment is completed at one appointment, has many advantages. It, however, may not be possible either because of time constraints, the difficulty of the case and/ or the expertise of the operator (dentist), or the severity of the infection. It is felt by some experts, however, that wherever practical, single-visit endodontic therapy is the more desirable way to go. A patient should therefore be able to discuss with the dentist during the examination stage if the root canal is one he can complete at one sitting. Note though that treatment outcomes are expectedly similar whether root canal treatment was done as multiple appointments or at one sitting.

Loss Of Turgidity and crowns

A root canal treated tooth can be likened to a plant. In plants there are channels from the roots to the branches right up to the leaves which carry food and water to all parts. This supply of nutrients, aside of providing nourishment, also keeps the plant turgid (strong) and sturdy. Hence, a plant devoid of such nutrients, wilts, loses its turgidity, becomes weakened and dies. Likewise, a tooth with its source of nutrients (the 'nerve') removed loses its turgidity, and is more brittle. Essentially, a root-canal-treated tooth is 'dead'. This phenomenon explains why the crown or the top part of a tooth so treated is thus weakened and will fracture more readily than a sound tooth. And it explains why you may be advised by your dentist after a root canal treatment to have the tooth capped or 'crowned', especially if more than half of the top part of the tooth is missing. And you guessed it, it may even be crowned with gold. What lucky tooth, the closest any joe bloke will ever come to feeling like the Queen of England—some excitement for a tooth, huh! This may probably be one reason root canals have become the most 'revered' treatment in dentistry.

It is not imperative that all root-canal-treated teeth should be crowned. Where a good part of the crown is intact (more than 3/4 is still standing) there may not be a need for a crown. A post may also be needed where more than half of the tooth crown (top part) is decayed off. In this case a pre-fabricated or a custom-made metal or plastic post will be inserted in the canal to strengthen the tooth and support the crown.

Aside of the future crown, the cost of a root canal depends on the number of 'nerve' canals in the particular tooth. Where it is a front tooth, which usually has a single root and therefore usually only one nerve canal, the fee is the minimum. The price jumps a little higher with two canals (or roots), and slightly higher in a three-rooted tooth with three or more canals. But mind you, a tooth with one root will not necessarily have only one canal, since some front teeth in the lower jaw may have two or more canals even though they may only have one root. Likewise, some back molar teeth have four 'nerve' canals even though they will possess only two or three roots. To each his own, as the saying goes.

There may be cases where the dentist will tell you he cannot fix a broken tooth, not even with a root canal. This is when the crown is severely decayed and fractured right down to the gum line so that there is not enough tooth structure or "collar" to hold on to at the gum line. At least 2mm of collar is needed above the gum line to provide support for the crown. Otherwise there will be leakage of saliva and other fluids down the tooth way down into the gums. The defective spot under the gum will start an infection in due course which may lead to the eventual loss of the tooth.

The other situation is where there is so much gum disease around the tooth that the tooth has lost much of its bone support, is not solid any more, and is now mobile.

'Capping' Or Crowning The Tooth

Sometimes a crown is the best treatment for a weakened tooth. A crown is just like a tight-fitting hat or 'cap' put on the tooth to cover and protect the weakened top portion. It should be made clear also that any tooth that has a lot of fillings or a very large filling (and is therefore a weakened tooth) is a good candidate for a crown. Hence, not only root-canal-treated teeth are destined to be Kings or Queens. Crowns come in different types, depending on the preference of the patient and the positioning of the tooth in the mouth.

The simplest, the 'stainless steel cap' may be prescribed in those cases where the individual cannot afford the real thing and wants the tooth saved for now until favourable financial environment prevails. This is of course less expensive and costs about 1/4 that of the gold crown. It is a pre-fabricated crown and comes in different sizes. The dentist will choose the one that just fits your tooth, trim it to accurately fit the tooth at the gum line and cement it on. This procedure only takes about twenty minutes.

The more expensive types are laboratory made. These may be of porcelain or metal or a combination of porcelain fused to metal. Here the tooth is prepared (cut down to size) by the dentist removing about 1.5mm of the enamel all around the crown of the tooth. An impression is taken of the prepared tooth and sent to the lab. An impression is made by taking the imprints of your teeth in a guey rubbery material in a fitted metal or acrylic container or tray. In the meanwhile the dentist will put a 'temporary' crown usually of acrylic material after the preparation of the tooth so as to prevent the tooth from becoming sensitive to temperature changes in the mouth. The whole procedure may take anywhere from an hour to two and a half. Hence, if you are going to have a crown prepared, you should not make a date or an appointment somewhere else in an hour's time. The dentist will feel rushed if you keep looking at your watch in between the various steps during the procedure and may not do his best job. Usually, you can allow a week to two weeks for the finished crown to come from the lab for it to be cemented on the tooth. These days crown fabrication is so fast you might get it the same day.

It should be cautioned that even though this type of crown is very hard and you cannot chew through it the porcelain crown can fracture with use. These days, this fracture can be repaired but it may leave a permanent fracture line so that the same area could fracture off again where the repair work is done right at the dental clinic. New products are on the market these days where the porcelain crowns, if made in the dental laboratories, are very hard and are said to be quite resistant to fracture. In the few cases that I have seen, a gold crown had been chewed through right to the prepared tooth. This may not happen if the owner has opposing natural teeth. In this case the owner had chewed through the gold crown because he had a false top denture (false teeth) which had been made of porcelain teeth and porcelain teeth can chew through the opposing metal crown with time.

A cast metal crown can either be of the non-precious variety in which case there is no gold in the alloy, or could be semi-precious with some gold content, and is of course slightly more expensive. It is, however, easier to chew through a stainless steel crown even when opposed by regular teeth since this crown is a lot softer than the laboratory-made cast types.

For those fortunate Kings and Queens, you can ask for your crown back should the capped tooth end up being removed as a result of a fracture or decay. I have heard it said that people have willed their capped teeth to beneficiaries on their death. I have even heard it said that 'people' (thieves) have exhumed and retrieved teeth from dead bodies for their crowns. Some respect for the dead, huh!

Pain and Root Canal Treatments

Pain experienced in a root canal treatment is usually postoperative, that is, often after the root canal procedure or in between appointments. As has already been mentioned, the main nerve bundles in the jaw shoot off branches to each tooth on its course along the jaw bone. Hence, each tooth is attached to its nerve supply at the end of the root, like a thread in a needle with the hole end of the needle representing the root end and the needle being the tooth. There is therefore a 'wound' of severed nerve end just at the root tip, with the remainder of the nerve supply represented by the thread at the needle hole. It is at this part of the root tip (the apex) where the postoperative endodontic pain (pain after the root canal procedure) originates. The root tip region (periapical or peri-radicular tissue — peri=round; radicular=of the root) becomes inflamed as a result of the wound in the area. Also, the cleaning of the whole length of the tooth right to the root tip (the filing and reaming by the dentist) may inadvertently force some debris (or 'detritus') down the root tip area. Pain may also be initiated as a result of some of the medications used in the treatment being forced into this root tip area. But despite all meticulous care during the cleaning and the shaping procedures, some periapical (peri=around; apical=of the apex or tip) inflammation may occur. But really, even the actual mechanical force exerted in the course of the cleaning of the canal may irritate the elements or fibers holding the tooth to the bone.

Not that this fact will console past or prospective root canal patients, but it has been found that approximately 40 to 57 per cent of patients undergoing root canal therapy will experience some postoperative discomfort; and that about 25 per cent may experience moderate to severe pain. The only use of this information is I suppose to give you more pain trying to determine beforehand if you are going to be one of the 57 per cent. Much good that will do you! Pain resulting from endodontic therapy may last from several hours to several days depending on the degree of tissue damage at the root tip and the extent of the inflammation (infection).

From the discussion above, it is logical to see that postoperative endodontic pain can therefore be reduced with the administration of anti-inflammatory medications. These could take the form of specific antibiotics where indicated or some appropriate anti-inflammatory painkillers. Aspirin, Tylenol and Ibuprofen have always been excellent choices in such cases. In situations where the pain is so intense or when the patient's reaction to pain is so exaggerated, a mood-altering drug may be called for. My only concern with these mood-altering drugs is that I fear these patients may really want to ride the beautiful pink elephants they imagine they are seeing while under the influence of these drugs. But these days there are some very good pain medications on the market to take care of any endodontic eventuality.

Finally, for those patients who grind their teeth a lot or who clench consciously or unconsciously, slightly taking down the crown on the tooth so that it is not hit while chewing may offer some interim relief.

Root Canals and Patient Communication

Dentists should be upfront with patients about the limitations of the root canal treatment. It is possible for the dentist to miss one of the 'nerve' canals in the tooth while the dentist searches to determine the number of canals the tooth has. For some reason I don't like telling a root canal patient at the outset about the effects of missing a canal. This information makes them more suspicious and will make many experience phantom pains even when there is none. But of course sometimes this un-cleaned canal will be the cause of the postoperative pain. If this is eventually identified it should be cleaned and filled like the others. And there will be an extra fee for this since there is a fee for each identified canal.

A dentist should be able to refer treatment (to the root canal specialist, the ENDODONTIST), if he finds the canals are more tortuous for his expertise.

The difficulty with root canals is that a small portion of them will cause problems in due course. I have seen a few instances where a root-canal-treated-tooth has had to be removed some years or even weeks later because of a flare up. Whether your particular treatment will be one of those that will flare up in the future is anyone's guess. But these possibilities should be mentioned to the patient, especially in the case of a badly abscessed tooth. The problem is that at the start it is impossible to determine how long this root canal will last before it may act up, because it may never act up again. If a problem is encountered during the process the patient should be advised and appropriate steps taken to remedy the situation.

Bleaching The Discoloured Tooth

You've been hit in a hockey game; or a horse kicks you in the mouth (as a farmer once told me); you have a car accident and you are lucky to get away with just a 'shaken, shocked' tooth which discolours with time; or you are plain socked in the teeth the last time you tangled with the in-laws. For some reason you have sustained a darkened tooth as a result. What will be your choice of a dental treatment? Or you get a root canal done and the tooth turns dark on you with time.

A live but discoloured tooth can be bleached just as a dead, darkened tooth. The bleaching techniques are a little different in the two cases but they are done everyday. The only downer (and really a small one) is that the teeth so treated tend to darken again anywhere from six months to a year's time and may have to be redone. Some of the methods used in dental offices these days to bleach the teeth have been shown not to present any problems. However, there are some on the market that you would want to check before using at home. From experience one is quite safe with the products (used by the dentist) that have been recommended by the Food and Drug Administration. The slight bleaching of the marginal gum area where some of the bleaching gel material inadvertently flows around the tooth at the gum-line goes away in a few hours without any subsequent trouble. There are some bleaching products, however that can cause problems like sensitivity of the teeth so ask your dentist.

CHAPTER 8

CROOKED TEETH, BRACES AND ORTHODONTIC WORK

You've probably seen those 'railway tires' (as young people 'favourably' call them) on people's teeth. You even see them on TV these days on the teeth of young actresses. They are metal wires going across the front teeth of usually people between the group of 12 to 18 years. These are called braces, and they are on the teeth for a very good reason — to straighten crooked teeth. There are many reasons why a reasonable human being will walk around with wires strapped across the teeth, and No, they are not Halloween RoboCop decorations. You would welcome one of these dental contraptions too if you had one of these conditions:

1. You happen to have crowded teeth. You were just lucky to have been born with a very small mouth so your friends cannot call you a big mouth. That is the good news. The bad news is that as a result of your good fortune to have avoided being branded a big mouth, now you do not have enough room in your head to contain all your adult 32 teeth within your little mouth. That means your top and or lower jaw bones are not large enough to have room for all your teeth. Hence the teeth are coming through any which way but straight. They may or may not look disfiguring and it may be your decision to seek a dental consultation.

2. You just happen to have inherited a lower jaw bone that is bigger than the top jaw bone. Some people have a more developed and pronounced lower jaw compared to the upper jaw so that the lower teeth (but especially the front teeth) find themselves sitting ahead and on top

of the upper front teeth. This condition is called PROGNATHISM and makes the top teeth sit inside of the lower front teeth while chewing.

On the average, most people have the lower front teeth sitting inside of the top front teeth. Look in the mirror right now and check your teeth. Bring your teeth together with the lower jaw moved as far BACK as you can move it back (this is called the Centric position). When in this position and for most people, the top teeth are 'slightly' ahead of and cover the bottom teeth. The operative word is 'slightly', because if the top front teeth are 'too far' out ahead of the lower teeth, this may be disfiguring and is called favourably by many people as 'bucked teeth'; 'anterior superior protrusion' or just simply a 'maxillary protrusion'.

The point to remember is that any difference from the subjectively 'ideal' bite is termed a 'Malocclusion; (mal = bad or occlusion = bite), meaning your jaws are poorly related, either the top jaw is bigger and hangs over the bottom jaw, or the lower jaw is ahead and in front of the top jaw. As you may have already deciphered, the basic problem with crooked teeth is really the relationship of the (top and bottom) jaw bones. The teeth just demonstrate the underlying poor jaw relationships.

Note that it may also happen that the jaw relationships could be right but the teeth positioning may not be ideal. This could lead to crowding of the teeth, especially in children, because—(1) someone neglected to fix the cavity in a baby tooth; the cavity got so big to the point where the tooth had to be removed; no spacer was placed in place of the baby tooth that was removed and so the new permanent tooth beneath could not find room in the jaw, causing crowding. (2) Or — someone simply neglected to have the cavity in the baby tooth fixed; as the cavity got bigger the adjacent teeth tilted or moved bodily into the space left open by the hole in the side of the decayed tooth, causing crowding. Otherwise in most cases of crowding the teeth are badly positioned because of poor jaw relationships.

Spacers and Space Maintenance

To understand the significance of the two statements above, let us tackle the question of space maintenance in the mouth. To put it simply, each of the 20 baby teeth in your 3-year old child's mouth will be systematically replaced by a second permanent tooth beneath it inside the jaw bone. These second set of teeth, the adult teeth, remain hidden inside the jaw bone until they are ready naturally to come into the mouth (erupt). As they begin to erupt into the mouth they cause the roots of the baby teeth, which all this time have been hiding and protecting the adult teeth, to dissolve away. Soon, the baby tooth begins to loosen and prepares to fall out (or exfoliate). The changing of the guards, á la Nature. Or as T.S. Elliot put it, "the old order changeth, yielding place to new".

Unless an x-ray reveals there is no permanent tooth under the baby tooth (i.e. no succedaneous replacement or the replacement is congenitally missing), the space occupied by each baby tooth needs to be carefully maintained, millimeter for millimeter, to preserve it for the new, soon–to-erupt adult tooth beneath it. The dentist will show you different types of appliances used to maintain the space should a baby tooth be removed or if lost prematurely (i.e. before it is naturally time for it to fall out). If no spacer is placed and there is a new tooth underneath the prematurely lost baby tooth there will not be enough room for the new permanent tooth, causing crowding in the mouth and probably a disfiguring of the child's teeth.

A little digression. As has been said, each baby tooth gets replaced by an adult 'permanent' tooth. If there is no adult second tooth to replace the baby tooth, then that adult tooth that did not form is said to be 'congenitally' (=from birth) missing. There are 20 baby teeth in all, and they account for 20 of the usual 32 adult teeth. Twelve more adult teeth come into the mouth or erupt in the adult to make the normal complement of 32 teeth. In some people, because the four wisdom teeth do not form or remain inside the jaw bone without ever erupting into the mouth, they end up having only 28 teeth. The adult 'permanent' teeth start erupting into the mouth as early as five to six years in most children, starting most of the time with the lower front teeth. In some societies (Ghana, West Africa) the lower front permanent teeth come into the mouth at the same time that the first permanent back molar teeth also show up in the mouth.

Does My Child Need Braces (Orthodontic Work)?

In many obvious cases parents know already that the child will need braces on account of the unmistakable crowding of the teeth.

What parents should remember though is that dentists are trained with certain 'norms and values' of the particular society and culture they practice in. For example, in North America, dentists are generally taught to close spaces between the teeth, especially open spaces (called 'diastema') between the top front teeth.

I remember as a young man in dental school in Canada, when this question came up in class—the treatment of the space in the upper two front teeth. I could not understand why the diastema needs to be closed up. This is because in my African society a space between the two upper front teeth is a sign of beauty and is sexy. Moreover, I was modeling a big gap of a diastema myself, and I could not see why I should have it closed and lose my one ace in the whole with which I hoped to actively attract members of the opposite sex. Of course no one was forcing me to close it but I now know why I had so much trouble getting dates! Back home the diastema is in such a fashion that people who have lost all their teeth for one reason or another and go to the dentist for false teeth would even ask for a gap to be created between the two front teeth. The diastema serves two purposes in any African society; aside of the attraction value, one can also make music with it by whistling through it. Can you hear me whistling?

Hence treatments are prescribed by dentists as a result of what they have been taught as 'normal' in the society. This issue becomes very ticklish when there is a border-line situation. Under these conditions, I suggest that parents go with their own 'feelings' and decide whether they want the treatment for their child. The reasons are twofold:

1. 'Braces' or orthodontic work, is a relatively expensive treatment. Especially where it is a border-line case and the family cannot afford the treatment. I feel the parents should not feel obliged Or the guilt that goes with refusing treatment, especially where the teeth positioning are not so bad as to be debilitating or be a handicap to the child. The dentist, as we expect from any competent dental professional, will draw your attention to any situation he recognizes in the mouth as 'abnormal' or to be outside the 'norm' as a result of his training. It is his duty as a clinician to tell you for fear that if he does not and you move away to another dentist or town, that some dentist will draw your attention to the state of the child's mouth and make him look incompetent. There are many occasions where a dentist will diagnose and tell you of a situation not to demand treatment but just to let you know that the situation exists. This precaution eliminates lawsuits and or the notion that the dentist does not know his work. Of course we hope that if it is a serious problem that he will insist you have it fixed. But once you the parent have been apprised of the situation you should then ask for an explanation as to any possible sequelae if the problem goes unfixed. With a lot of these orthodontic border-line cases, there are many people walking around with these conditions who don't feel handicapped. In fact in my practice, I would usually call the parents aside after my examination and discuss with them my findings if I felt the condition to be quite acceptable without braces. But I do NOT discuss the findings in front of the child patient. My reasoning is that especially if the condition has not up till now been seen to be a problem, I do not want to "label" the child and now create a monster. Young people are very impressionable and all the dentist needs to do is talk about a malocclusion or that the bite is bad and the youngster goes around with a complex. If no one in the family has recognized a problem in the youth's bite, but especially if the youngster has hitherto not seen any problem with his/her bite, I would mention the existence of this mild malocclusion to the parents but will let sleeping dogs lie, as the saying goes. My philosophy is, as is with most people, 'if it ain't broke, don't fix it". Of course if the parents decide to have the mild condition treated, sure, it gets fixed.

But the message here is that if you the parent(s) size up the diagnosed condition and feel it is mild and acceptable enough to leave without treatment, you should listen to your instincts and not forever have that guilt hanging over your head as if you've let your child down. I have children too and we all want the best for our children. However, if a condition, especially some mild orthodontic 'problem', is unearthed and it can be accepted, do accept it and move on to the next more pressing item on the agenda. I have seen too many parents who, from all indications, cannot afford an orthodontic treatment, and one that would not make too much of a difference in the child's appearance, but have forever felt guilty and down-trodden over it because the dentist said it should be fixed.

We have to make choices in this world and there are priorities; what would you do if your only family car (for a family of four) is on its last legs and you have $4000 saved and you realized that your daughter would need an orthodontic treatment costing $4000? If you felt that the child's facial appearance was quite acceptable even though your dentist says it should be done, what would you do? There is no question what I would do and it does not for a minute mean I don't love my children. I am stressing this point because I have seen too many parents distressed and agonizing over this issue. It goes to show that beauty is indeed in the eye of the beholder. Perfection may not necessarily be what one needs in life and may not be what you need to fulfil your destiny in life. Ain't that the truth!.

Adult Braces

These days orthodontic work is for everybody—no matter what age group. If you missed having your teeth straightened when you were a child you can now have it done, and yes, even at fifty years old. You see, now, if you cannot afford to give your child perfectly straight teeth you can ask him/her to wait and have it done later on in life when there is a little more cash in the till, hopefully. But remember that it would take a little longer time to complete such treatments in the adult because of the thicker and more matured bone density.

Also, some needed treatment in the adult may demand that only one or two teeth be moved with braces. For example, where a tooth which is to be used as an anchor for a bridge is tilted badly, braces may be recommended to straighten the tilted tooth before it can be utilized for the bridge support (bridge is discussed later).

And then to weight-watchers. I have received not a few requests from patients who want braces but for weight reduction. In this case, although the treatment may look like orthodontic braces, the teeth are actually wired together shut for some time. People got this idea from the fact that individuals involved in an accident and have sustained broken jaws usually have their jaws wired shut to prevent movement of the broken parts in-order to promote fast and proper healing.

But, hey, to each his/her own, and if you want your teeth wired to close the trap that is always demanding, "feed me, feed me", all power to you. But something tells me this route will not work because just like the child who has an orthodontic appliance placed to prevent the habit of thumb-and finger-sucking but who eventually finds a way around the appliance in order to continue the sucking, the individual so wired will find a way, when there is the will, to "feed" the habit. I can imagine one Monday morning such a patient walking into the dentist's office with a mouth full of broken, tangled wires. Reason? Over the weekend there was this scrumptious barbecue she could not refuse and had the spouse or the next door neighbour put his pair of pliers to the dentist's deft handiwork so she could partake of the feast.

Whether it is in an adult or a young person, these braces have to be kept spectacularly clean every day. They have to be kept clean and you have to clean them not just every day, but after each meal. Otherwise the wires would certainly trap food or collect food particles which would rot your teeth. You can use a toothbrush and toothpaste or any cleaning brush your orthodontist will give you; but whatever you use, please keep those teeth and wires cleaned.

I have seen some young people, and I must admit a very few, who never even returned to the orthodontist to remove the wires at the end of treatment and came to have them removed four years later. You can guess in what state the teeth and wires were, especially since the wires were to have been removed in a year and a half or at most in two years.

CHAPTER 9

FALSE TEETH. 'DENTURE', 'PLATES' OR FALSIES

It appears some people are still queasy about false teeth. I don't know whether it is because they are afraid of it or because they are disgusted by it. But I have heard of people who will not drink out of a glass when they visit any friend who wears false teeth just because at one time they found one of their friends keeping her teeth in a glass of water. This may be a strange reaction to one incident but it goes to show you how queasy some people are with false teeth (or 'dentures'). And then there are those who wonder how it would be like to kiss someone with false teeth. It is smooth, let me tell you. (I bet you are wondering if I have tried it!!!). The only advice I can give you is if you are one of the queasy types then take good care of your teeth, else you will not only be keeping one in your glass but will be drinking through one before you know it.

It is not too difficult to get yourself in a position where you will be a candidate for a set of choppers. We see the ingredients every day in the dental office. All you need to do to wear one of these, are :

1. not to brush teeth and gums everyday (at least once);
2. eat a lot of sugary, sticky foods especially in between meals;
3. neglect to have your gums and teeth properly checked and cleaned at the dentist's (at least once a year);
4. neglect to have cavities fixed.

But for some unlucky individuals doing all the right things may still land them in denture-land (the land of the tooth-fairy) if they get into an accident like playing NHL or Pee-Wee hockey, a car accident or if they happen to keep horses and they get socked in the mouth by one of their own horses. Some payback for your kindness, huh!

Interestingly, I know of people who proudly profess never to have brushed their teeth after they turned thirty and still have all their teeth at age sixty-five. Why the cut-off point at thirty and not twenty-nine, I don't know but you don't try to copy them. Testing mother nature this way, (and why do we say mother nature and not father nature, anyway?) may just be your ticket to the Never-Ever Land of Denturedom. You may be the unlucky bloke who will find that in his forties the teeth keep falling out one by one for no apparent reason, to you anyway.

Why False Teeth, You Ask

There are many reasons why people wear dentures.
1. **Neglect**
2. **Accidents**
3. **Mental sickness**—it may shock you to learn that in some societies people with mental problems who are difficult to control have all their teeth taken out. Either because they will not need them to eat (ha!) since they are fed pap anyway, or else to prevent them from ever again biting those trying to hold them down to take their teeth out. Poetic justice huh!
4. **Personal wish.** Some people just get tired taking care of their teeth and decide to bid them adieu. Good riddance. That's the way to do it —as the bible says, when your eye is bothering you, pluck it out; when your teeth are bugging you, just pull them out. That will fix them. Sometimes I wonder if taking the teeth out for false teeth isn't changing one problem for another. But so far it seems to work for the advocates of this exchange program. If you make up your mind to go toothless you somehow look at the exchange in a positive mode and it will then work for you, I suppose.

5. **Old Age**—you do not necessarily have to wear false teeth just because you are old. And at what age can we legitimately say one is 'old' anyway? But gum disease tends to be more predominant as we age, and those more susceptible to gum disease may lose their teeth as they get older. Now, if you ask me if a forty year old individual is 'old', I will say not yet. Is a seventy year old, 'old'? Maybe. I guess so, according to the Bible, anyway— that God has given us to live "three scores and ten". After that, hmm, you are just damn lucky! But something tells me though that if one has been taking particularly good care of one's teeth throughout, that the chances of one losing one's teeth are infinitesimally small all the way to old age.

6. **Natural Disaster**—some individuals may have the misfortune of being born with a variety of dental malformations which may demand expensive cosmetic dentistry. Some may also have had a variety of childhood sicknesses as a direct result of which treatment would render the teeth unsightly. Problems like hypo-calcification (improper hardening of the teeth from poor calcium utilization), amelogenesis imperfecta (poor enamel formation, the outside layer of the visible parts of the teeth) and tetracycline stains (discolouration of the teeth as a result of taking tetracycline antibiotics while a child for the treatment of some sickness) fall in this category. In such cases lack of funds for expensive cosmetic work on the natural teeth may give way to choosing the less 'expensive' (financially, anyway) alternative of removing all the teeth and inserting false teeth.

Going For False Teeth

If you decide on false teeth when you have already lost all your natural teeth you simply visit the dentist and you will be fitted with one. At the first appointment the dentist will study the shape of the jaw bones which will be the supporting structures for the new (false, mind you) teeth. Any special features of the mouth will be noted in order to produce a fitting denture. For example, if the bony ridges are very sharp he may require some surgery to smoothen and attempt to remodel the top of these ridges so as not to cause pain when you bite with the plates. Also, some people have bulbous bony protruberances on the side of their jaw bones (called 'torus' or 'tori=plural). These tori, more prevalent in the lower jaw, will interfere with the proper seating of the plate and may have to be removed and bone remodeled. If one has been gumming it for a long period of time the bony ridges, through natural process of resorption (loss of the top layer of the jaw bone), become very flat. This condition presents the most difficult case to treat and is the dentist's nightmare. It is difficult at this stage to tell the patient that the plates may not fit tight. How do you explain to someone that the new false teeth will not fit tight when you've just been asked to promise to make a denture with 'a good fit'?

The Need For Implants

To the dentist a good fitting denture is a term with quite a different connotation from what a patient would call 'a good fit'. To the dentist a good fitting denture could still float in the mouth and rock and roll, given a flat jaw bone, as long as the impression is accurate and the teeth fit into each other without interferences while in function (i.e while it is being used, like eating or talking). To the patient, however, a good fit means a tight-fitting set of choppers, one you can only remove with a pair of pliers. Because of poor fit the only satisfying solution for some patients will be to have 'implants'. With (false-teeth) implants the denture base fits securely into metal 'posts' or 'plates' anchored or 'implanted' into the jaw bone. Hence the false teeth can sit rigidly on even a flat jaw held in place by metal posts sunk into the jawbone.

Implants can be used to rehabilitate (treat) the completely edentulous (toothless) mouth or the partially edentulous (mouth with some teeth). There are different types:

Type 1: immediate— Implant post and tooth are placed same day in same area where tooth was removed.

Type 2: where the metal posts and plates Are placed inside the jaw bone and left for about 2 to 4 months to allow healing of the supporting gums and bone before adding on the top teeth.

But implants are not for anyone, either. One has to be in good health, must be willing to devote time to the proper cleaning process and must have some money (may cost from $6,000 onwards per denture, the cost of course depending upon the number of missing teeth to be replaced. One woman I know spent $30,000 for her full set of upper and lower implanted teeth). An implant candidate should not be one who habitually grinds or clenches the teeth. One should also be patient and must commit to the multiple visits to the dentist since the surgical preparation before fitting the false teeth in some cases may take weeks or months to make sure the surgical sites have healed well. For those who can tolerate regular dentures it is just as well because implants will not be for you. But for others who can't wear or don't like to wear the conventional denture and can afford it, implants can make a dramatic difference.

The Fabrication Of False Teeth

You will want to discuss the fees for the set of false teeth even before the impressions are taken. The fee quoted usually includes any necessary adjustments after delivery (or insertion) up to three months from the date of insertion. There are usually anywhere from two to three appointments to complete the fabrication of a set of dentures (a set being the two, top and bottom). Initial study impressions are taken; then a second more accurate impression with the bites taken and size and colour of teeth selected, and then a try-in stage to see if the teeth arrangement is acceptable. These models made from the impression then are sent to the dental laboratory for processing and finishing. Then, the last appointment is more for delivery of the teeth to the patient (insertion stage). This may be the last appointment and for some patients it is the last they see of the dentist.

But it is advisable to return to the dentist for a check in the first week even when there is nothing bothering you. Sometimes certain spots under the plates will alert the dentist of possible sore spots. All these potential sore and trouble spots can be relieved before they become seriously handicapping. And let me tell you, some denture soreness, especially where a flange (the sides touching the cheek or the tongue), cuts into these areas, can be so excruciatingly painful that it makes some big men cry. One gentleman described it as a 'toothache'. And yet it takes only a few minutes for the dentist to relieve the extended flange or border and bring instant relief. A lot of patients do not come in to have these problems fixed and instead just chuck the false teeth and return to gumming it, a very unnecessary, wasteful and expensive gesture.

Immediate Dentures

You may, however, have some natural teeth still in the mouth and for one reason or another may decide to have them all removed and be fitted instead with false teeth. These are what dentists call 'immediate' dentures. Most dentists in this day and age will not subscribe to this idea and will try to talk you out of it. I remember for one patient of mine I stalled and stalled and stalled. Like Penelope in Illiad's story of Odyssey, I would make the first impression one day only to tell the patient the next appointment that I had misplaced the previous impression. I would take another only to misplace it the next appointment. He must have thought I had the most disorganized franchise going but he faithfully stuck with me, nevertheless.

(For those who do not know who Penelope was, she was in Greek mythology the wife of Odyssey, the King of Ithaca who, as a punishment from the gods, was kept at sea for ten years because he had conquered in battle a favourite town belonging to the gods. During the absence of the husband the King, Penelope, because she was very beautiful Queen, attracted a lot of suitors in her courtyard. The most tormenting part of her ordeal was the fact that each of these unscrupulous suitors wanted to be King and replace Odyssey, her husband. These men therefore all came to live in her palace and daily harassed her to choose one of them for a husband. But Penelope, beleaguered as she was, was a very loving and faithful woman and believed her husband would return one day (call it a woman's intuition). So, she made a pact with the suitors that she was going to weave a tunic and on the day of the completion of this tunic she would choose one of the suitors for a husband. Each day the men would see her busily at work with her weaving, all the while taunting her to hurry it up. But what they did not know was that each night Penelope would meticulously unravel what weaving she did that day. The next morning she would be at her weaving again in full view of all. Then, that night she would painstakingly and again unravel all she had done that day. To cut a long story short, she was right and was able, with this wisdom and cunning, to stall the suitors until the eventual return of her husband ten years later).

In this one case I think I made about four (primary, initial, or study) mouth impressions until I was very convinced from his tenacity that the patient really wanted this done and nothing would sway him from this intent. I had wanted to wait him out, hoping that with time something would make him change his mind and decide to retain or keep and fix the remaining teeth instead.

There are two methods generally employed by dentists in the fabrication of an immediate complete denture and you will be asked to choose the technique you favour.

In one technique the few remaining teeth are removed first and the gums are given time to heal before the false teeth are made. The time allowance will vary anywhere from two weeks to three months, depending on how fast the patient wants it and the condition of the mouth. In my experience, the average waiting period has been about two weeks. Not too many people want to go toothless for too long, for obvious reasons. In some cases they only have two weeks before their daughter's wedding in which case one week of waiting is all they get. However, where the teeth are in a bad shape, for example in the presence of a severe periodontal (gum and bone) disease, I would usually try to bargain for a little longer waiting period to allow the ensuing more extensive shrinkage of the gums to occur before making the dentures.

Where the second technique is preferred, (and lots more patients go for this method, again for obvious reasons), the false teeth are first made. When the dentures come from the dental laboratory and are ready in the dental office the natural teeth are then removed and the plates inserted the same day, i.e. right after the extractions (teeth removal). This procedure is faster but presents a few more problems; it also demands some patience on the part of both the dentist and the patient because multiple visits may be needed for subsequent adjustments. There is also some soreness, especially in the lower jaw. Eating offers a slight problem because you will be chomping over a fresh wound so the patient tends to go on a diet 'á la hospital' — just mush. Then, as the days go by and the extraction sites start to heal the gums all don't heal at the same rate. Different parts of the mouth heal at different rates and so the plates also tend to fit differently at different times. This process causes soreness in different areas at different times and will have to be relieved for comfort.

Usually with an immediate denture where this second technique is used one is supposed to leave the false teeth in the mouth for the first day without any attempt to remove them. If you dare remove them sooner for some reason, often the swelling after the surgery and the pain will prevent you from being able to reinsert the teeth. A few times this happened I had to scrape a lot out from inside of the denture and make it bigger to fit it. And then, the denture now becomes too big so I next had to reline the inside with a soft liner to make it fit tighter and more comfortably.

If the new teeth are left in the mouth for the required twenty four hours after the extractions, the teeth can then be removed and cleaned the next day. The mouth is then rinsed with some warm salt water (a glass of warm water with a half teaspoon of the common table salt) or with some mouthwash if the taste and / or the smell is abominable, and this is usually the case at this time. From here on one is advised to keep rinsing with salt water as often as is possible, say once every two hours.

In most provinces in Canada the cost of the immediate denture usually includes three months of adjustments as well and patients are usually advised to use this time to have all necessary adjustments made before this time of limitation. Technically, every adjustment made after the three months can be charged for, although in many offices adjustments are made for free as long as the work was done in that office.

Lining The Denture

Especially with an immediate denture, the need will usually arise where they have to be relined ('lined') on the inside to fill in where the gums have shrunk during the healing process. During the initial three months soft liners are intermittently employed whenever needed. The patient will know when a new soft lining is needed by the fact that either the lining material deteriorates and becomes hard and rough or the plates gradually become loose. In practice, I found that within the first few months of fabrication that I have had to reline or adjust new immediate dentures about every three weeks to a month.

It is at this stage that a lot of misunderstanding appears on the scene, and it is either due to poor communication or else the patients were told but did not 'hear' because it was a future event and did not want to bother with details better left for when the time came. And the problem has to do with the 'permanent' reline. Permanent relines attract a separate fee and is not included in the initial fees for the false teeth. However, even when patients are initially told that they would have to pay extra for the subsequent 'permanent' reline that may be needed some time later after the three to six months grace, they always manage to forget and bicker about this fee. If you are having problems in this area the trick is to write the agreement in the chart and let the patient sign that the permanent reline would attract an extra fee.

Other consideration will have to be made at this time as well in relation to doing the reline. The 'permanent' reline can be done right in the dental office in which case the patient gets to go home wearing the dentures. The other way where the false teeth are sent to the dental laboratory for the reline means the patient goes for a few days, in the rural areas for two days, without the teeth. I never liked doing these 'final' relines in the office because I did not like the finished product. The reline comes out OK but I could never finish the plates as nice as I wanted and I always, told the patients that. Where they did not mind and planned to shut themselves up in the house for the duration of the two days and did not mind the risk of going out and being seen toothless, the relining was sent to the laboratory for processing. But whenever it was impossible to part with the teeth for no matter how long, arrangements were made with the laboratory so that the patients went personally to the laboratory and had the reline done that same day while they waited.

How To Take Care Of Your False Teeth

Your work is not over just because you have a set of dentures. They still have to be cleaned just as when you had your natural teeth. I guess if you ever brushed your natural teeth you could extend the same favour to your false teeth. But if you now want to turn over a new leaf, you may start by brushing your 'falsies' using a toothbrush; yes, the same instrument you never wanted to see again. It is the same thing over again. Toothbrush and some toothpaste or soap are all you need for this chore.

It is recommended that while cleaning the teeth, this time around having the easy task of holding them in your hands, that you have some water in the sink or over a bowl over which you will be doing the scrubbing. This way the water in the sink will break the fall should the teeth slip off your hands.

Dentists have generally been taught to ask patients to take the dentures out at night and store them in a cup (or a glass) of water. The reasoning is to allow the gums which have been under immense pressure all day long to now relax and take a breather. You would too if you were subjected to the kind of forces and pressures exerted on you every day during the chewing process. You can use a glass of water but be careful not to use the same glass while offering your visitor something to drink. That will probably be the last you see of him. There are specially made denture 'baths' which you can obtain from your dentist or probably from the drug store for this purpose.

The only problem I have with this recommendation of taking the false teeth out at night is that you may have a few patients, especially women, in my experience, who may not relish the idea of taking the teeth out of their mouth AT NO TIME, no how. A few women have actually revealed to me their husbands don't even know they wear false teeth! Poor guy, I wonder what he thought the smooth gums were! Some smooth woman you've got! Now the cat is out of the bag. But please don't go fishing around trying to determine if your wife is wearing a set of falsies. For the sake of these few individuals who want to play hide-and-go-seek, I feel the rules can be bent a bit. I feel these individuals can be asked to wear their teeth at night (otherwise you the dentist may be sued for 'alienation of affection', now how about them apples?), but should try to take them out of the mouth whenever the husband is out of the house, like say when he is in the bathroom? Especially if he is like me who spends hours there in the toilet reading Prevention, Readers' digest or the Dental Journal.

I cannot for the life of me understand how little people know of dentistry or teeth, especially when the profession has been around in North America for at least two centuries. It appears a lot of people get their dental information from their friends or neighbours or relatives; warmed over and 'cooked information' and very inaccurate at that. For example, why should one feel that because 'a friend' has been wearing dentures for twenty years and has not had any adjustment all these years should therefore imply that you would and should also have the same experience? This reference is so irrelevant that when a patient quotes me such statistics about their friends or a neighbour or a relative I always marvel how people can think like that in such an information-laden environment. But then this is why I am writing this book. Another statement commonly made about immediate dentures: a friend of mine says he never had to reline his (immediate) dentures from the day he had them and he has had it for five years now. To that I say, all power to him.

The comparison appears incomprehensible to me because North America is supposed to be a place where people want to be treated as people, individually and not grouped into mere numbers. People take pride in being themselves. People want to be treated as unique individuals. But what these denture wearers are doing, tells me they are gradually losing their individuality and are grouping themselves into masses of non-entities. They are behaving as if their bodies are identical to their neighbour's or 'friend' or relatives'. Otherwise why would they want their bodies to behave exactly as their 'friends"? It is almost futile for the dentist to answer. "But your mouth is not the same as your friend's. You are you and your experiences are going to be different from your neighbours, believe it or not". They've been functioning under this false comparison mode for so long that half the time they don't believe the dentist who says, sure, your friend may not have needed any adjustments but you may because you are different. The unfortunate aspect of this belief is that such patients believe they need adjustments because you did not make good dentures for them.

Dentures should be checked whenever they fit differently and start hurting. They may need relining or rebasing if they appear to be too loose in comparison to how they fit previously. If it hurts because it is cutting some part of the gum or is ulcerating an area, this can be relieved in a few minutes. If they are cracked or broken they can easily be repaired in a few hours. Denture problems should never be postponed, although many refuse to have them checked until they get so bad they cannot wear them any longer.

The funny thing about false teeth is that if they are bothering you because of a high spot somewhere or because it is too tight in another place, it will never go away until the offending area has been relieved. You can put all kinds of salves, powders or adhesives in the plate and it won't make a difference. Until the particular spot is relieved it well keep coming back to haunt you.

A lot of denture wearers believe that nothing needs be done on their dentures once they've had them; that they should be good for ever and there should be no need for any adjustments. People do not appreciate that there is bone under the gums and so the gums and the underlying bone support the dentures. With time therefore the gums undergo changes. As a result the plate, dentures or falsies made to fit the mouth at one point in time, will need to be adjusted to fit the bone as it undergoes these inevitable changes. Hence, adjustments should be done whenever needed. It is a wonder how resilient humans are. Sometimes, you see a set of dentures that you know are just floating around in the mouth. You attempt to remove the lower plate and the top plate unhesitatingly falls out with it. They are so loose you wonder how they stay in the mouth. And yet, when you ask the owner how the plates are you are met with the answer. "Oh, Great!. I have had no problems with them all these thirty years". Thirty years and he has not had any problems. Impossible! A lot from this generation (I mean sixty years, and over) have been under the false impression that a denture needs no adjustments and that they are good for life. They feel that when you have problems with them it is time for new ones, and since they can't afford new ones, they have to make these do.

As a result a lot go around with ill-fitting dentures and do not seek advice. They feel it is supposed to be that way. And then there are those who just chuck the dentures and go without when it starts bothering them either because they say they don't want to bother the dentist or they decide the dentures 'don't fit' and were not 'made right'. I know people with three sets of dentures all made in the space of one year and do not think of going to the dentists who made these in order to make them fit comfortably; shows you how tolerant people can be if they have to.

PROLOGUE

SEXUAL ABUSE AND THE "POWER OF IMBALANCE" IN DENTISTRY

Now, can a dentist treat his own wife?

I had to address this issue since I read about a ban on dentists treating their spouses as instituted by the Ontario and British Columbia Dental Associations in Canada. I wonder what has happened to this decision presently although I know it is still in the books. I have never been able to understand this law and thought it had something to do with the Combines Act or some kind of a Competition Act in relation to monopoly. But I found out I was wrong and it had nothing to do with competition. For example, I also thought that they may want to put a stop to the practice of a dentist working on his own wife for the obvious feeling that a couple can plan and deliberately charge fees for work not done. After all who else gets into the spouse's mouth?

But NO, that is not the reason! HOW WOULD YOU FEEL IF YOU WERE A DENTIST AND WERE TOLD YOU COULD NOT DO ANY DENTAL WORK ON YOUR WIFE BECAUSE YOU COULD BE CHARGED WITH SEXUAL ABUSE? Now wouldn't this ruling be enough to make anyone crazy? Not that dentists are clamouring to work on their spouses. In fact I can imagine many trying to avoid having to work on their wives. But I could not find reasons for this crazy ruling until I later learned it was a law passed not specifically against dentists but against all health professionals who would also treat their wives as patients.

Somewhere in the Health Professions Procedural Code "sexual abuse" is defined as sexual intercourse or other forms of physical sexual relations between the member (eg dentist or physician) and the patient. This therefore obviously includes spousal relations if your spouse happens to be your patient. The very controversial "dentist/spousal patient ban" still exists because the law makers do not want to make any exceptions for the sake of preserving unanimity in its application.

The rationale for this ruling is that the health professional is in a higher power situation, as they put it, and that "power imbalance" exists in such a relationship. This is incredibly unfathomable, because such an "imbalanced" relationship can be found in many life situations. Isn't there, for example, a 'power imbalance' in a taxi driver / passenger relationship? The ruling is so absurd that somewhere in the explanation they now have added that there has to be "active treatment". Now what is "active" treatment? I guess as long as the dental work is going on? So the spouse ceases to be a 'patient' and sexual relations can resume when the fillings are all done, until the next appointment time or the next recall annual check-up? Boy, that is interesting—so you stop having sexual relations with your wife whilst she is under 'active treatment', for say a month, then you resume sexual activity during the hiatus of the following eleven months? Actually, that is not too bad. Some couples have less activity than this and one month of abstention in the year is really not bad. In fact if I was younger I would use this technique as my birth control strategy. Roman Catholic dentists, here is one way to beat the system.

But there are other puzzling questions:

a. will the dentist be charged with sexual abuse if the dentist happens to be a woman with a male husband patient? For example, will the female dental hygienist be charged for cleaning her husband's teeth (now who says women can't take the initiative, huh)? I would love to see that.

b. Will the dentist be charged if his spouse who is also a patient is another man? And how about a female dentist with a female spouse patient?

c. I can imagine a scorned or aggrieved wife reporting or suing the dentist husband for sexual abuse just to get back at him. Ordinarily though the defence of "consent" should definitely apply in all these cases. I admonish dentists therefore not to take X'rays or keep a chart, essentially not leave any kind of a paper trail of any sort when treating the spouse. And also to work without an assistant in order not to have a witness. Wow...

The dental student and patient relationships

The resultant implications, however, differ for the dentist versus the dental student. The student is not in a position of power imbalance, not yet anyway, until he becomes a doctor. It may not land the student in court for sexual abuse but it may have even more serious consequences.

This topic is very dear to my heart because it almost cost me my dental degree. You see, as a dental student and especially in the final two years to graduation, you are supposed to complete a certain number of treatment requirements to show you are competent enough to be released onto the unsuspecting population. But no one warned me to stay away from the practice of using your girlfriend as patient whilst you are still a student. Funny, huh, because you can't treat your spouse when you are a dentist or your girlfriend when you are a dental student.

I saw this knockout of a girl assisting the Oral Surgery lecturer in one of our classes and Oh, she was fine, well built with some heavy looking behinds that would put even the Kardashians to shame. I did not know the Kardashians then, of course, (this was in 1971) but this young nursing assistant would've compared quite favourably with any woman on earth, bum for bum. So we became very good friends, and became an "item" or began "dating" as they used to say in the 70s.

Now in the final year of dental school I had to complete a "bridge" as one of the treatment requirements. To require a "bridge" one would have lost one or any number of teeth in the mouth thus creating a space somewhere in the mouth. This space though has to have a tooth ahead of it and another tooth behind it. With one or more teeth ahead and behind the space you then construct a bridge where false teeth are joined to the adjoining teeth on each side of the space.

My girl and I were doing fine until I got this 'brilliant' idea of bringing her into the clinic as my bridge patient. Now maybe I should've been warned not to treat my own girlfriend but I was having problems getting a suitable bridge patient for the class and felt this was an arrangement made from heaven. As a dental student I felt 'big' and proud playing doctor treating my girl, coupled with the fact that the work would cost her very little since it would only cost her the price of the gold that I would use in fabricating the bridge. You see, in dental school those days the student fabricated everything himself and did all the lab work as well. It would also close the big gap in the middle on the left side of her mouth when she smiled. It was a 4-unit bridge. So she was missing two teeth in the middle and the tooth on each side of the space would be used to support the two teeth we would be replacing. So it was all good, right? WRONGGG!

Like I said, everything was going on swimmingly until she (my girl) saw me one day driving another woman's car with the other lady in the car! I had purchased some $500 rickety old VW but she did not see me driving my VW. At least I would've probably had some good excuse. I was driving this lady in the lady's own car. Now that was inexcusable!

You see, I was a foreign student on scholarship for Dentistry in Canada. Back in my country in Africa I had girlfriends, sometimes even two simultaneously but there was no problem. Of course there, no one would have ever seen me driving another woman or her car. I had no car, and none of the girls I had had cars either. Hence it would only be hearsay and I could defend myself nicely even when caught.

I did not know there was a problem until the bridge clinic came up and all my classmates were well into their cases. I had no patient but of course I told my supervisor that oh my girlfriend is coming. If the supervisor knew something I did not know and he never let on. I am sure it must have happened before where the 'date' patient did not show so mine could not have been the first time. Moreover, a few of my classmates were working on their girlfriends too. What I wasn't privy to was the fact that maybe these Canadian mates knew the rules of engagement and knew how to treat their women who were also patients.

An hour passed and the two-hour clinic was half done and still no patient. So I called her on the clinic phone. At the other end of the line issued some vituperations I cannot even repeat. And I had to watch my words or cover my hand over the mouthpiece because the telephone was the clinic phone and the receptionist could hear all the conversation. But no, it was not a conversation! Oh, she was angry. Then she told me, that she had seen me driving with another woman.

To cut a long story short, we completed the bridge but not without some gnashing of teeth on my part in the three months it took to complete the work. Suffice to say that when she was in a good mood she showed up. If not, she did not come in, but she had to have it done because the temporary bridge she had on her teeth were not the greatest or hottest piece of work. I had smartened up with advice from one of my mates to make sure the temporary bridge I fabricated should not look good, even though it would fetch me low marks for lousy work. (We had to put in a temporary bridge whilst working on the final bridge in the lab). But I eventually did make up with a pretty decent finished bridge which fetched me a more than passing mark because it was a long and involved bridge. To the dental student, however, a divorce would have been probably more acceptable than failing your final year graduating examination.

And you think I would learn from all this? Oh NO. In the final year in the same class of restorative dentistry I had this young 18 year-old girl who had about seven amalgam (the gray) fillings in her mouth that I had done. Again, in those days in the 70s, a filling was not complete for grading by the Prof unless it has been polished beautifully, smooth and shiny. Now here I was, with an appreciable amount of amalgam fillings in this girl's mouth and the darn girl would not come in for polishing so I could get my marks to graduate. So what did Ishmael Bruce do? (And mind you, I got this idea from the same mischievous class mate who gave me the idea of the not-so-nice temporary bridge). I got this idea, therefore, to date this girl on the weekends to keep her buttered up and put her in an amicable and pliable position to come for her Monday appointments. So I would obediently take this girl to the movies on the weekends in order to keep her amicable enough for her Monday morning appointments. Oh, what I wouldn't do for a buck! And that explains why I was so broke especially in my final year of dental school. And maybe that explains now why I was caught with a girl in the car. Oh no—I was not caught 'with a girl in the car'… I was caught 'driving with a girl in the car'. Kapish? So for you all dental students and dentists, watch who you date or marry. It just may come back to haunt you. And coming to think of it, wouldn't such harrowing experiences in four years of dental school make anyone crazy? Well, I rest my case.

USEFUL REFERENCES

1. Selden et al, 2000;
2. Touyz, Louis Z. G: The Acidity (pH) And Buffering Capacity Of Canadian Fruit Juice And Dental Implications; J Can Dent Assoc 60: 1994
3. Kleemola-Kujala, E. and Rasanen, L.: Relationship Of Oral Hygiene And Sugar Consumption To Risk Of Caries In Children. Community Dentistry And Oral Epidemiology 10: 224-233, 1982.
4. Moss, Stephen J: Growing Up Cavity Free; A Parent's Guide To Prevention. Quintessence Publishing Co. Inc. 1993.
5. Report Of The Working Group On Preventive Dental Services: Preventive Dental Services; Practices, Guidelines And Recommendations. Health and Welfare Canada, 1979.
6. Bruce, Ishmael: Epidemiological Aspects of Developing a Preventive Dental Strategy for Canadians. Thesis presented towards Master of Science Degree in Public Health Dentistry, University of Toronto, Canada. 1986.
7. Early Childhood Caries the Leading Cause of Day Surgery for Canadian Children. Website: cihi.ca

Printed in the United States
By Bookmasters